ETHICS AND RESEARCH ON HUMAN SUBJECTS

INTERNATIONAL GUIDELINES

Proceedings of the XXVIth CIOMS Conference
Geneva, Switzerland
5-7 February 1992

Edited by Z. Bankowski & R.J. Levine

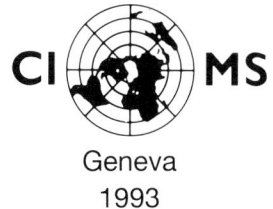

CI MS

Geneva
1993

CONFERENCE PROGRAMME COMMITTEE

Bankowski, Z. Secretary-General, Council for International Organizations of Medical Sciences (CIOMS), Geneva, Switzerland

Bryant, J.H. Professor, Department of Community Health Sciences, The Aga Khan University, Karachi, Pakistan; Co-Chairman of Conference

Dickens, B.M. Professor, Faculty of Law, University of Toronto, Toronto, Canada

Gutteridge, F. Consultant, Council for International Organizations of Medical Sciences (CIOMS), Geneva, Switzerland

Heymann, D.L. Chief, Office of Research, Global Programme on AIDS, World Health Organization, Geneva, Switzerland

Levine, R.J. Professor, Yale University School of Medicine, New Haven, Connecticut, U.S.A.; Co-Chairman of Conference

Reprinted 1993

Copyright © 1993 by the Council for International Organizations
of Medical Sciences (CIOMS)
ISBN 92 9036 054 2

TABLE OF CONTENTS

ACKNOWLEDGEMENTS

The Council for International Organizations of Medical Sciences (CIOMS) acknowledges the very substantial contribution, financial and technical, of the World Health Organization Global Programme on AIDS to the preparation of the International Ethical Guidelines for Research Involving Human Subjects, and of the Conference on Ethics and Research on Human Subjects — International Guidelines, of which this volume constitutes the proceedings. The two other Special Programmes of the World Health Organization — on Research, Development, and Research Training in Human Reproduction, and for Research and Training in Tropical Diseases — also gave valuable support. CIOMS acknowledges also with much appreciation the financial contributions of the Sandoz Foundation in the United States of America and the International Development Research Centre of Canada.

Of the many individuals who contributed to the success of the Conference and the preparation of the Guidelines, the following merit special acknowledgement: Professor Robert J. Levine who was Co-Chairman of the CIOMS Steering Committee and of the Conference on Ethics and Research on Human Subjects — International Guidelines, and provided invaluable assistance from the inception of the project, particularly in the preparation of the several drafts and the final text of the Guidelines; Professor John H. Bryant who co-chaired the Conference and the Steering Committee; and whose wise counsel was available throughout; Professor Bernard M. Dickens and Mr. Richard Kelly who prepared the first draft of the Guidelines; Professor Lawrence O. Gostin, for his part in preparing An Annotated Guide to Ethical Review, which was used in the preparation of the Guidelines; Professors Mohamed Abdussalam, Wendy Mariner and Benjamin O. Osuntokun, Mr. Frank Gutteridge, Mr. Sev S. Fluss and Dr Michel Thuriaux, who contributed actively from the beginning; and the authors of the conference papers, and the moderators and rapporteurs of the three conference working groups. Special thanks go to Dr James Gallagher for his contribution to the final drafting and editing of the Guidelines and the editing of the Conference proceedings, to Mrs. Kathryn Chalaby-Amsler for her invaluable secretarial help and her part in the organization and management of the Conference and the Steering Committee meetings, and to Mrs. C. Dübendorfer for her secretarial assistance in connection with the Conference.

INTRODUCTION

Conferences of the Council for International Organizations of Medical Sciences (CIOMS) are designed as international and interdisciplinary forums in which scientists as well as lay people can exchange views on topics of immediate concern, unhampered by administrative, political or other considerations. They are intended especially for the discussion of the scientific and technical bases of advances in biology and medicine and other related areas, as well as their social, economic, ethical, administrative and legal implications.

Advances in biomedical science and technology, and their application in the practice of medicine, are provoking some anxiety among the public and confronting society with new ethical problems. Society is expressing concern about what it fears would be abuses in scientific investigation and biomedical technology. This is under-standable in view of the methodology of biomedical experimental research. Investigation begins with the construction of hypotheses and these are then tested in laboratories and with experimental animals. For the findings to be clinically useful, experiments must be performed on human subjects, and, even though carefully designed, such research entails some risk to the subjects. This risk is justified not by any personal benefit to the researcher or the research institution, but rather by its benefit to the human subjects involved, and its potential contribution to human knowledge, to the relief of suffering or to the prolongation of life.

Society devises measures to protect against possible abuses. The first international code of ethics for research involving human subjects — the Nuremberg Code — was a response to the atrocities committed by Nazi research physicians during the second world war, revealed at the Nuremberg War Crimes Trials. Thus it was to prevent any repetition by physicians of such attacks on the rights and welfare of human beings that human-research ethics came into being. The Nuremberg Code, issued in 1947, laid down the standards for carrying out human experimentation, emphasizing the subject's voluntary consent. In 1964 the World Medical Association took an important step further to reassure society: it adopted the Declaration of Helsinki, most recently revised in 1989, which lays down ethical guidelines for research involving human subjects. In 1966 the United Nations General Assembly adopted the International Covenant on Civil and Political Rights, which entered into force in 1976, and which states (Article 7): *"No one shall be subjected to torture or to cruel, inhuman or degrading treatment or punishment. In particular, no one shall be subjected without his free consent to medical or scientific experimenta-tion"*. It is through this statement that society expresses the fundamental human value that is held to govern all research involving human subjects — the protection of the rights and welfare of all human subjects of scientific experimentation.

In the late 1970s, in view of the special circumstances of developing countries in regard to the applicability of the Nuremberg Code and the Declaration of Helsinki, CIOMS and the World Health Organization (WHO) undertook a further examination of these matters and in 1982 issued *Proposed International Guidelines for Biomedical Research Involving Human Subjects.* The purpose of the *Guidelines* was to indicate how the ethical principles that should guide the conduct of biomedical research involving human subjects, as set forth in the Declaration of Helsinki, could be effectively applied, particularly in developing countries, given their socioeconomic circumstances, laws and regulations, and executive and administrative arrangements.

Proposed Guidelines received wide distribution and, according to a later survey, went into use throughout the world, providing valuable ethical guidance in biomedical research involving human subjects. Survey respondents and other users indicated also that the guidelines should be reviewed with particular reference to the ethical issues raised by large-scale trials of vaccines and drugs, transnational research, and experimentation involving vulnerable poulation groups. A particular indication for their revision was the prospect of field trials of vaccines and drugs to control AIDS. Moreover, in recent years, many people, in developed and developing countries alike, have begun to see research involving human subjects as beneficial and not only threatening, and indeed such research, particularly therapeutic trials, is now actively sought by potential beneficiaries. For some, participation in research is the only way they can gain access to valuable new treatment or even general medical care; for others, it is the means by which scientists will discover new knowledge that may lead to the prevention or treatment or even elimination of certain categories of disease and disability.

In these circumstances CIOMS undertook, in collaboration with WHO, the revision of the guidelines, setting up a steering committee to guide the process. The Steering Committee decided that in the revision special attention should be paid to epidemiological studies, owing to the importance of epidemiology, particularly for public health, and to the lack of international guidelines for ethical review of such studies. In the event, it was determined that the need for epidemiological ethical guidelines would be best met by a separate publication, and the result was the issuing by CIOMS in 1991 of *International Guidelines for Ethical Review of Epidemiological Studies.* The preparation of the epidemiology guidelines contributed materially to the revision of the 1982 guidelines.

After extensive consultation the first draft of the revised guidelines was prepared by a group of consultants, reviewed and amended by the Steering Committee, and presented to the CIOMS Conference on

Ethics and Research on Human Subjects — International Guidelines, held in Geneva in February 1992, of which the proceedings are contained in this volume. At the conference it was examined and discussed by some 150 participants from both developed and developing countries, including representatives of ministries of health and of medical and other health-related disciplines, health policy-makers, ethicists, philosophers and lawyers.

The primary themes of the conference were:

- *Consent of individuals and agreement of communities to participation in research*, including concepts of consent and the communication to prospective research-subjects of information to enable them to give valid informed consent, inducements to consent, selection of subjects, special concerns of disadvantaged or vulnerable populations, and problems of fully informing and gaining the agreement of communities.

- *Ethical review processes*, such as national and local committees, practical impediments to ethical review, review of externally-sponsored research, and developing the ethical-review capacity of host countries.

- *Obligations of sponsors*, with special attention to responsibility for access of subjects to medical services, access to beneficial results of research, care and compensation for injury resulting from research, and development of the research capacity of host countries.

In addition, there was discussion on emerging issues in resarch, such as the effects of different cultural concepts of ethical principles and values on the conduct of multinational research, challenges to the application of ethical principles in particular research areas such as HIV infection, the influence of ethical principles and guidelines on legislation, and the ethics of research into the human genome.

The three primary themes and the additional topics were explored in plenary presentations and discussed in working groups. A special plenary session was devoted to different cultural perspectives on ethics and research involving human subjects.

The draft guidelines were revised to reflect the consensus of the conference, but with due regard to minority points of view. The revised draft was sent for comment to the conference participants, to international associations, and to medical research councils and other interested bodies and institutions in both developed and developing countries. The final text duly reflects the comments received. It has been endorsed by the WHO Global Advisory Committee on Health Research and the Executive Committee of CIOMS.

The text, which is included with the conference proceedings in this volume and also published separately, consists of a statement of general ethical principles, a preamble and 15 guidelines, with an introduction, and a brief account of earlier international ethical declarations and guidelines. Each guideline is followed by a commentary.

The guidelines reflect the paramount ethical concern for vigilance in protecting the rights and welfare of research subjects and of vulnerable individuals or groups being considered as prospective subjects. Like the original (1982) guidelines, the revised guidelines are designed to be of use, particularly to developing countries, in defining national policies on the ethics of biomedical research, applying ethical standards in local circumstances, and establishing or redefining adequate mechanisms for ethical review of research involving human subjects.

Certain areas of research do not receive special mention in these guidelines; they include human genetic research, embryo and fetal research, and fetal tissue research. These represent research areas in rapid evolution and in various respects controversial. The Steering Committee considered that since there is not universal agreement on all the ethical issues raised by these research areas it would be premature to try to cover them in the present guidelines.

The mere formulation of ethical guidelines for biomedical research involving human subjects will hardly resolve all the moral doubts that can arise in association with such research, but the guidelines can at least draw the attention of investigators, sponsors and ethical review committees to the need to consider carefully the ethical implications of research protocols and the conduct of research, and thus conduce to high scientific and ethical standards of research.

Zbigniew Bankowski, M.D.
Secretary-General, CIOMS

OPENING OF THE CONFERENCE

F. Vilardell
President, Council for International Organizations of Medical Sciences

Dr Jardel, Assistant Director-General, representing Dr Nakajima, Director-General of the World Health Organization, Members of CIOMS, Distinguished Guests, Ladies and Gentlemen.

As President of CIOMS it is for me a great privilege to welcome you all to the XXVIth CIOMS Conference, in which the draft CIOMS International Guidelines for Biomedical Research Involving Human Subjects will be revised. As you already know, the first version of these guidelines was published in 1982. Since that time there has been clearly a need to review some aspects of the guidelines.

I should like, in the first place, to thank Dr Nakajima and WHO for making this Conference possible. WHO has always been of great help to CIOMS in its undertakings to provide the medical world with a forum for the discussion of the many vitally important issues in the fields of ethics, medical educaton, taxonomy and nomenclature of diseases, technology transfer, health policy-making and medical sociology.

This is probably the most important CIOMS Conference since the publication of the 1982 Guidelines, and the culmination of our programme on ethical guidelines. It is hoped that during the next three days many of you will participate in the discussions and support the Steering Committee in finalizing this revised edition, which, I am sure, will be of great help all around the world, but especially in countries where a bioethical awakening and consciousness is taking place.

May I thank the members of the Steering Committee for their performance of the arduous task of preparing the materials which will be discussed here, the chairmen of the Conference — Professors Bryant and Levine, and Professor Dickens who kindly prepared the background discussion paper.

I now have the honour of introducing Dr Jardel, Assistant Director-General of the World Health Organization.

J.-P. Jardel
Assistant Director-General, World Health Organization

Mr. President of CIOMS, Professor Vilardell,
Mr. Secretary-General,
Messrs. Co-Chairmen,
Distinguished Guests and Colleagues,
Ladies and Gentlemen.

The Director-General of the World Health Organization, Dr Hiroshi Nakajima, absent from Geneva, has asked me to represent him today at the beginning of this important Conference. It is therefore my privilege to welcome you to WHO headquarters, and to wish you every success in your deliberations, which are anticipated with great interest by the Organization.

Our particular focus in this last decade before the year 2000 is on public health. The cornerstone of our action remains the achievement of the goal of Health for All by the Year 2000. However, this by no means implies a lack of interest in advances in medicine and medical progress in general. As stated by one of the promoters of the 1982 Proposed International Guidelines, the late Dr Norman Howard-Jones: "... human experimentation is the *sine qua non* of medical progress." These words highlight the importance of this Conference, and WHO wishes to assure you of its continuing support.

Both WHO and CIOMS have played an important role in disseminating the Proposed International Guidelines for Biomedical Research Involving Human Subjects, which emerged from the series of international conferences sponsored by CIOMS during the period 1978-1981. And yet we are aware of continuing problems in the implementation of these Guidelines at national and, even more, at local levels. We are all aware of the rapid advances in biomedical research, and the emerging new areas that are being addressed by investigators in developed and developing countries alike. If one examines the agenda for the XVth Round Table Conference, held in Manila in September 1981, and the impressive agenda that Dr Bankowski and his colleagues on the Organizing Committee for this Conference have prepared, one sees how far we have come in a decade.

In this connection, allow me to say how pleased I am to see the continuity that has guided CIOMS in selecting the key architects of the draft International Ethical Guidelines for Biomedical Research Involving Human Subjects. I hope that all of you will contribute to the debate on this draft and guide CIOMS in its further development and refinement. All of us welcome particularly the participation of experts from developing countries, who I am sure will greatly enrich the coming discussions.

There is one final point I should like to make, and that is the growing importance of ethics and human rights in health care in general, and in biomedical research in particular. The human-rights and ethical dimensions are gradually coming to the forefront of our activities. We count on the strong support of CIOMS to provide us with guidance and counsel as these activities develop over the coming years. We are aware of the very important programme entitled Health Policy, Ethics and Human Values — an International Dialogue, which CIOMS launched some years ago and whose Steering Committee is chaired with dynamism and imagination by Professor Jack Bryant.

Permit me to end by quoting from Elie Wiesel, winner of the Nobel Peace Prize, who has stated:

"... respect for human rights in human experimentation demands that we see persons as unique, as ends in themselves."

This concise yet lucid formulation will, I am sure, be at the very centre of your debates.

KEYNOTE ADDRESS

Robert J. Levine
Professor of Medicine, Yale University School of Medicine, New Haven, Connecticut, U.S.A.

This Conference is convened at a pivotal point in the preparation by CIOMS of *International Ethical Guidelines for Biomedical Research Involving Human Subjects*. We have before us a draft of the revision of the 1982 Guidelines. Now we suspend the writing to have this consultation, to review what has been accomplished and to seek consensus on what remains to be done. We have the good fortune to have assembled at this meeting a diverse group of distinguished experts who have demonstrated their commitment to developing guidelines for the ethical conduct of research involving human subjects around the world. Many of them have participated in the process of revising the 1982 Guidelines since it began; indeed several were participants in the conferences that informed the development of the original document.

No longer "Proposed"

The proper title of the 1982 Guidelines is *Proposed International Guidelines for Biomedical Research Involving Human Subjects*. Some readers have assumed that because they were called "proposed" their authors considered them incomplete or perhaps a semi-final draft; this is incorrect. The 1982 Guidelines were a finished product in all relevant senses of the word. They were called "proposed" because they were intended as a proposal to various agencies that had the authority to make and, if necessary, to enforce biomedical research policy — such agencies as governments, academic and professional societies and institutions, and research-based pharmaceutical companies. In the decade since they were promulgated, they have been influential in guiding the ethical conduct of research involving human subjects.

The central purpose of the 1982 Guidelines was to provide a detailed interpretation of the Declaration of Helsinki to facilitate the correct application of its principles. There was particular concern with the need to provide guidance for research initiated or sponsored by agencies in developed countries and conducted in developing 'host' countries; this continues to be a major objective. The revised document will also recognize that similar problems may arise when research is conducted in developing communities within developed countries.

Protectionism

In common with all international codes of research ethics and virtually all national legislation and regulation in this field, the 1982 Guidelines project an attitude of protectionism. The dominant concern in such documents is to protect individuals from injury and exploitation by the relatively much more powerful scientists and physicians. Indeed, when the United States first promulgated federal regulations in this field, it entitled them "Policy for the Protection of Human Research Subjects" and assigned responsibility for assuring compliance with them to the "Office for Protection from Research Risks."

In his classical essay, *Philosophical Reflections on Experimenting with Human Subjects*, Hans Jonas wrote of "conscripting" subjects to "sacrifice" themselves in the "service of the collective"; his was an accurate portrait of the prevailing attitude of the 1960s. In 1966 the United Nations General Assembly adopted the International Covenant on Civil and Political Rights, of which Article 7 states: "No one shall be subjected to torture or to cruel, inhuman or degrading treatment or punishment. In particular, no one shall be subjected without his free consent to medical or scientific experimentation." Thus biomedical research was regarded as an enterprise related to torture or to cruel, inhuman or degrading treatment.

There are important historical reasons for such images so to have dominated scholarly commentary on, and public attitudes about, biomedical research and focused concern of the drafters of ethical codes and regulations on the need for protecting the rights and welfare of human research subjects. The first international code of ethics for research involving human subjects, the Nuremberg Code, was drafted in response to evidence given at the Nuremberg War Crimes Trials of atrocities committed by Nazi research physicians. Many of their experiments had entailed the deliberate killing of, or infliction of grievous injuries on, prisoners, whose rights to consent or refuse were ignored. Thus, the field of research ethics began as a search for secure defences against repetition of the most egregious assaults on the rights and welfare of human beings ever committed in the name of science.

The perception of research as perilous was reinforced by news of the Thalidomide disaster and, in the United States, by exposés of research activities in which the standards of Nuremberg and Helsinki were or appeared to have been violated. Public reaction to the Tuskegee syphilis studies, the Willowbrook hepatitis studies and other similar cases led directly to the legislation that established the National Commission for the Protection of Human Subjects of Biomedical and Behavioral Research and charged it to identify the basic ethical principles that should underlie the conduct of research involving human subjects. The principles identified in 1976 by the National Commission — respect for persons, beneficence, and justice — have since found their way into international documents, including the draft of the revision of the 1982 Guidelines, which is the centrepiece of the agenda of this Conference.

I do not mean to suggest that the early ethical codes ignored the fact that research could be beneficial as well as threatening. The

Nuremberg Code recognized, indeed required, that research "should be such as to yield fruitful results for the good of society." The fruitful results, however, were not featured so prominently as were the threats to the subjects. Rather, they were seen as constraints on the amount of threat to the subject's well-being that would be tolerated: "The degree of risk... should never exceed that determined by the humanitarian importance of the problem to be solved."

Revisionism

In the decade since the 1982 Guidelines appeared it has become increasingly apparent that many people have come to regard research involving human subjects as beneficial. Some see participation in research as the only way they can gain access to valuable new therapies. For others it is the only way to secure access to general medical care. Some groups of people value participation in research because it is the only way information can be developed that will lead to improved therapies for members of their groups.

What has caused this change of perspective on research? Even in the 1950s and 1960s there were those who recognized that some participants in research regarded their participation as beneficial, but the message began to become increasingly clear early in the 1980s. When Dr Barney Clark received the first artificial heart, many commentators — academics and journalists alike — were saying "Isn't it wonderful that this man, so near the end of his life, is willing to sacrifice himself in the service of other people." According to the psychiatrists who were in close contact with Dr Clark, however, it is very clear that he saw the artificial heart as the only way to pursue his survival. The only alternative was certain death. He stated most poignantly how upsetting it was for him to be unable to finish combing his hair, because even this slight exertion made him desperately short of breath. While he acknowledged that he would be pleased if others could profit from his experience, this was clearly not his primary objective.

The message became even more clear later in the 1980s, during the placebo-controlled trials of AZT in the treatment of patients with AIDS. Now we began to hear a new voice — the very articulate and increasingly powerful voice of the AIDS activists. They correctly pointed out that enrolment in this clinical trial was the only way to get even a 50% chance of receiving the only therapy that offered any hope of delaying death or the onset of opportunistic infections. The widely held perception among persons with AIDS that participation in this clinical trial was much more a benefit than a burden was so powerful that some patients even faked the inclusion criteria to be included in this clinical trial. The perception of this drug as valuable was so strong, even among physicians, that some primary care physicians cooperated with patients in falsifying inclusion criteria.

6

Thus, in remarkably short time, the prevailing image of research has changed dramatically. Investigational drugs, once regarded as dangerous 'Thalidomides,' are now described as 'promising new therapies', access to which should not be denied to persons with serious illnesses. People are now demanding access to randomized clinical trials, previously regarded as experiments in which persons were stripped of the 'good of personal care' and treated as 'statistical objects'. The principle of justice, which requires equitability in the distribution of both burdens and benefits, provided the philosophical grounding in the 1970s for protecting vulnerable persons from bearing the burdens of participation in research; now it is invoked to assure equitable access to the benefits of participation in research and of promising investigational therapies. The pendulum has come full swing. I believe that the current tendency to see research as largely beneficial and benign is just as erroneous as the earlier tendency to view it as primarily dangerous and exploitative. The revised Guidelines should present a balanced perspective, reflecting the need to encourage the conduct of ethical research while maintaining necessary vigilance to safeguard the rights and welfare of research subjects.

Avoiding overprotection

The revised Guidelines should reflect our recognition that policies designed to protect vulnerable individuals from bearing the burdens of research may inadvertently create barriers to the development of therapies essential to combating their diseases. Policies designed to protect children, for example, resulted in making them, in the words of the paediatrician, Harry Shirkey, "the therapeutic orphans of our expanding pharmacopoeia." Such deprivation of vulnerable populations of the benefits of new diagnostic, preventive and therapeutic products should be recognized as a class injustice. The revised Guidelines should not erect unjustified obstacles to the involvement in research of children or of persons with disabilities attributable to mental or behavioral disorders or to intellectual or psychological impairments.

All women, and particularly those to whom researchers and their sponsors commonly refer as being 'of childbearing years' or 'biologically capable of conception', have inappropriately and unwillingly been labelled vulnerable. Consequently, along with children, they have been susceptible to being 'protected to death'. The revised Guidelines should be responsive to their rightful insistence that they be included as subjects of biomedical research.

In passing, it is worth noticing that some nations have responded to the changed perception of investigational new therapies for serious diseases by adopting policies to facilitate access to these 'promising new therapies' even during the conduct of clinical trials designed to evaluate their safety and efficacy. In the United States we call such policies 'expanded access' and 'parallel track'. Such policies designed to facilitate early access to promising new therapies should not arbitrarily exclude either women or persons properly identified as vulnerable.

HIV infection and AIDS

Many of these changed perceptions of biomedical research and its ethics have been shaped in response to HIV infection, to AIDS as a disease and to the AIDS pandemic as a social phenomenon. It is not so much that AIDS has presented us with unique or unprecedented ethical problems: rather, it has forced us to pay attention to problems that were there all along. In retrospect, we notice that we should have addressed them earlier.

In the autumn of 1991 newspapers around the world reported that four countries had been identified as likely sites for clinical trials of candidate vaccines for HIV infection — Rwanda, Uganda, Thailand and Brazil. Many people reacted to this news with concern: Will there be meticulous review by research ethics committees in these countries? Will it be possible to get adequate informed consent? Is the motivation to reduce costs by exploiting persons in developing countries to develop products intended only for the lucrative markets of developed countries? These are the sorts of questions that those newspaper reports elicited. They were asked in letters to the editors of newspapers and of professional scientific journals. Just a few days after the announcement they were also asked at a meeting of the United States National Institutes of Health AIDS Program Advisory Committee. These questions symbolize another reason for revising the 1982 Guidelines now: AIDS has heightened our awareness of the necessity to conduct in developing countries research initiated in technologically developed countries.

The role of the WHO Global Programme on AIDS

The time was ripe for a revision of the 1982 Guidelines but it was the needs of the WHO Global Programme on AIDS (GPA) in connection with the field testing of candidate HIV vaccines which precipitated the decision of CIOMS to initiate the revision. In 1990 a GPA consultation on criteria for international testing of candidate HIV vaccines raised the subject of ethical, social and legal issues, and GPA therefore decided to prepare a comprehensive document on the matter. Wendy Mariner and I were assigned to draft guidelines for the development not only of candidate vaccines but also of drugs for HIV infection. The document we produced consisted of a detailed interpretation of the CIOMS 1982 Guidelines designed to cover the various contingencies we anticipated in the development of drugs and vaccines for HIV infection. It was necessary, of course, to incorporate some provisions more or less specifically directed at the field of HIV infection. More importantly, we also found it necessary to introduce some substantial revisions in the provisions of the 1982 Guidelines — revisions of the sort I have mentioned earlier. It was apparent that some of the revisions we were proposing were equally relevant to research in other fields. For this reason it was agreed that it would make more sense to undertake the revision of the 1982 Guidelines than to develop a document limited to HIV infection.

Unresolved problems

As we prepare to take the next step in revising the Guidelines, it is necessary to attempt resolution of some difficult problems, which, for purposes of this Conference, are arranged in three categories: informed consent, ethical review procedures, and obligations of sponsors.

After we have discussed each of these topics in plenary sessions, we shall divide into three working groups, each of which has been assigned questions in one of these three categories. The working groups are to focus their attention on these questions as they arise in the conduct of research initiated in or sponsored by a developed country but conducted in a developing host country or in a developing community within a developed country.

Here are some examples of the difficult questions we shall address:

In communities in which individual informed consent is incompatible with cultural traditions, to what extent can one rely on consent by community leaders? How can one be confident of the legitimacy of the leaders' authority?

In communities in which the right of women to be self-determining is not acknowledged, can their participation in research be authorized? If so, how?

How and by whom can one be authorized to conduct biomedical research in communities in which the concepts of scientific medicine and research are not well understood?

How can one assess the legitimacy of material inducements to participate in research? Is there a level at which they become 'undue inducements'?

What does it mean to require that the ethical standards applied in a host country should be no less exacting than they would be for research in the initiating country? Does it mean that the procedures should be the same or that the guiding principles should be the same?

How can one assure that externally sponsored research is appropriate in the light of national and community priorities within the host country?

To what extent should sponsors be expected or required to provide assistance, financial, educational and other, for the development of scientific and ethical review committees: and to make the drugs, devices and vaccines developed reasonably available to subjects, communities or nations afterwards?

To what extent should sponsors be expected or required to provide health-care facilities? Should these be made available to all members of the community in which the research is conducted — not just those who consent to participate? Should these facilities be maintained by the sponsor after the research programme has been completed?

These and other questions prepared by the Steering Committee will be presented to the working groups. I hope that as a result of their reports and other discussions at this Conference we shall be able to develop guidelines that are as satisfactory and timely in 1992 as the 1982 guidelines were a decade earlier.

INTRODUCTION TO THE DRAFT REVISED GUIDELINES

Bernard M. Dickens*

Introduction

Momentum for reform of the CIOMS 1982 Proposed International Guidelines for Biomedical Research Involving Human Subjects was deliberately initiated by CIOMS almost immediately on their release a decade ago. Responses were actively sought to the Guidelines from many agencies representing the biomedical research community they were designed to affect. The purpose was not only to acquire short-term evaluation of their contents and anticipated consequences, but also to accumulate material on their long-term effects in use. The present exercise to revise them may be seen not necessarily as corrective of errors or inadequacies in the 1982 Guidelines, but as a step in their anticipated evolution. To serve its role, CIOMS aims to be alert to evolving values, perceptions and circumstances in research relevant to the medical sciences, and to update its guidelines accordingly.

Although the 1982 Guidelines addressed ethical concerns that investigators are expected to consider, a wider intended readership has to be recognized. Lay (meaning non-biomedically qualified) members of committees that prospectively review proposals for biomedical research on ethical grounds have become more numerous, in part perhaps because of the emphasis the Guidelines gave to the need for such committees. Such members require easy access to ethical guidelines that investigators have to observe, and the CIOMS Guidelines were intended to serve their requirements as well as those of investigators. In addition, members of different national publics, including governmental officers, journalists and commentators who inform and may represent such publics, appear increasingly concerned with the ethical guidelines according to which biomedical research is planned, approved, funded and executed.

A decade of general development in the critical environment of biomedical research has compelled reconsideration of the 1982 Guidelines. In addition, however, a number of specific new circumstances have shown a need for more refinement of detail than the early guidelines offered, of which human-immunodeficiency-virus (HIV) infection and the related acquired-immune-deficiency syndrome (AIDS) are the most obvious. A number of these specific developments will be identified below, following consideration of the need to make explicit the underlying ethical principles of the Guidelines.

* Faculty of Law, Faculty of Medicine and Centre for Bioethics, University of Toronto, Toronto, Canada.

Ethical principles

The Guidelines that CIOMS widely distributed in 1982 had been endorsed by the CIOMS Executive Committee in September 1982 and by the World Health Organization's Advisory Committee on Medical Research in October 1981. Their preparation began in 1976, however, when CIOMS and WHO initiated a collaborative project. At that time, such documents as the 1947 Nuremberg Code and the 1964 World Medical Association's Declaration of Helsinki, as amended in 1975, were available as guides to medical research. These codes of conduct addressed such issues of continuing concern as research subjects' free and informed consent to participation in research, and observance of scientific principles in the design and execution of studies. However, their focus on correct conduct left implicit the underlying ethical principles to which the rules of conduct gave effect — that is, the codes that guided investigators' attention and practices were silent on the ethical values and principles that inspired the details of the guidance offered. The 1982 Guidelines similarly left concealed the ethical foundations on which their specific provisions were constructed.

It is considered that the revised Guidelines should make their underlying ethical principles explicit. The field of moral philosophy, from which such principles are drawn, historically influenced by cultural, political and religious values, is not so cohesive or coherent that principles can be expressed that are universally agreed, interpreted or prioritized. The principles that come most readily to the minds of many leading activists in the development of research guidelines, the so-called "Belmont principles," disclose their own cultural and related origins in the traditions of Western Europe and modern North America. It is a continuing topic of discussion and controversy whether the Belmont principles are also found, as many claim, in the traditions of other cultures, such as those of the Islamic world, sub-Saharan Africa, South-East Asia and China.

The Belmont Report, which articulated the principles, officially entitled *Ethical Principles and Guidelines for the Protection of Human Subjects of Research*, was developed by the United States National Commission for the Protection of Human Subjects of Biomedical and Behavioral Research, from discussions held in February 1976 at the Smithsonian Institution's Belmont Conference Center, and issued in 1979. The Report was published through the U.S. Department of Health, Education and Welfare (now the Department of Health and Human Services). The Commission was assisted by scholars from the Kennedy Institute of Ethics, at Georgetown University in Washington, D.C., and the principles are sometimes described as "the Georgetown principles"; indeed, they are now so frequently recited in bioethical discourse and analysis, by no means limited to the ethics of biomedical research with human subjects, that they are also referred to jocularly as "the Belmont mantra."

The ethical principles are respect for persons, beneficence and justice. Respect for persons includes the two sub-principles of autonomy of persons capable of meaningful or rational self-determination, and protection of the personal and psychological integrity and the dignity of those who are not capable of autonomy. The principle of Beneficence, meaning the duty to do good, is often taken to include the ethic of non-maleficence, the duty to do no harm, which has been basic to medical care since before the time of Hippocrates. The ethical principle of Justice, which includes the duty to treat like cases alike, is the principle to which the law is devoted, but not to the exclusion of other agencies or processes.

The level at which the ethical principles are applied is a matter of particular concern to the revision of the 1982 Guidelines. Although practices have evolved in many Western and Westernized cultures to prioritize individualism, for instance over collectivism, and therefore to apply ethical principles at the person-to-person (or microethical) level, the principles accommodated at their conceptual origins an application at the group-to-group and group-to-individual (or macroethical) levels. A clinical study that an investigator undertakes on a subject will implicate ethical principles at the microethical level, but studies addressed to populations as such, as opposed to each individual within the population, will implicate principles applied macroethically. Revision of the 1982 Guidelines was initiated at the time when CIOMS was actively preparing guidelines for epidemiological studies. The CIOMS 1991 International Guidelines for Ethical Review of Epidemiological Studies are intended to influence preparation of the revised Guidelines, and emphasize the collective or macroethical application of respect for persons, autonomy and, for instance, non-maleficence.

Epidemiology was addressed in the 1982 Guidelines, but without the depth and refinement that has subsequently become appropriate. Other factors that have led to and conditioned the revision process also merit mention.

Factors conditioning revision

AIDS and HIV infection. The WHO Global Programme on AIDS influenced the conclusion by CIOMS that the time had come to prepare a revision of the 1982 Guidelines. The AIDS pandemic has had many effects on the practice and perception of biomedical research on human subjects, at national, international and international-organizational levels. At the level of practice, the relatively short times between diagnosis of HIV infection, onset of AIDS, development of full-blown AIDS and death, perhaps with dementia intervening in later stages of the infection, make it ethically imperative to accelerate or put on a "fast track" many drug and vaccine studies that offer some prospect of assisting sufferers, without compromising the studies' scientific or ethical propriety. Further, the sense of urgency that HIV infection has produced has led to innovative research techniques, including community-based studies and high levels of community participation in the design and execution of studies. At the level of perception, HIV infection has created a demand that biomedical research be undertaken and a perception that such research is beneficial to persons included as subjects. Its obstruction or delay is accordingly seen as maleficent. This counters the long-prevailing predominant perception stemming from the post-1945 Nuremberg War Crimes Trials that medical research is prone to victimize its subjects and treat them merely as human guinea-pigs.

Population studies. In addition to inducing developments in clinical drug and vaccine research, HIV infection has widened recognition of the need for epidemiological studies, to determine the prevalence of disease among members of a given population. Epidemiology, meaning literally the study of epidemics, is a study technique employed by many health scientists, such as pharmacologists, who would not consider themselves to be epidemiologists. Further, some who do describe themselves as professional epidemiologists consider that they are practitioners and not researchers. For these reasons, the 1991 CIOMS International Guidelines for Ethical Review of Epidemiological Studies are directed to the conduct of epidemiology as such rather than only to professional epidemiologists, and to studies in general rather than to research as distinct from practice. For purposes of the revision of the 1982 Guidelines, however, it is intended to cover only epidemiological research.

Studies of population groups to determine the prevalence of pathological conditions raise ethical issues even when not concerned with conditions as sensitive as HIV infection. Although such studies are properly described as concerning collectivities of individuals and not identifiable persons as such, they clearly implicate and may affect persons as individuals, and personal identities may become known to investigators. This is less likely to happen when studies deal with anonymous medical data or surplus samples of body tissues, such as blood, that cannot be linked, or that cannot be linked other than through extraordinary effort, to their human sources. When identifiable medical records are involved, however, concerns arise at both macroethical and microethical levels of assessment.

Investigators in epidemiology are entitled to their boast that evidence indicates that they maintain fastidious standards of confidentiality. Nevertheless, their claim that they stand within the charmed circle of persons entitled to access to medical data from identifiable individuals who have not explicitly approved their access in advance needs to be reviewed independently in each case. The

14

revised CIOMS Guidelines recognize that the application of ethical rules may have somewhat different outcomes in public health studies from outcomes reached in clinical studies. The priority that the value of autonomy has achieved in the emphasis given to subjects' autonomy in clinical research may be displaced in public health studies by such values as protection of vulnerable persons and beneficence. Information about pending studies may be given, for example, through news media and other publicity, and consent may be inferred from passive silence rather than be sought by explicit affirmation.

Development of the 1991 CIOMS Guidelines for epidemiological studies generated the sense that the 1982 formulation should be reconsidered in light of the distinction between applying ethical principles in clinical studies and applying them in studies pitched primarily at a population-based or macroethical level. Different strategies from those relevant to clinical studies may have to be developed to respect the autonomy of population groups, and to protect groups against violation, indignity and risk of harm. Concepts of consent, confidentiality, protection and compensation for injury may have different implications at different levels of application.

Environmental concerns. Transcending macroethical concerns are those that arise from studies that may produce ecological or environmental consequences, seen in the broadest sense. It may not at first appear likely that research with human subjects will have such consequences or risks, although clinical studies to prevent or relieve human infertility may quickly be related to the environmental consequences, in a particular country and beyond, of high rates of human reproduction. Similarly, studies designed to limit unplanned pregnancies and to afford women enhanced means of personal self-determination may affect the balance of authority within a community, and its agricultural, economic and social practices. Both clinical and public health research have had effects of an environmental nature — for instance, concerning the composition of human diets and the adjustment of food production to meet new patterns of consumption.

The revised 1982 Guidelines will have been achieved through collaboration of persons sensitive to the wider and long-term foreseeable effects of, for instance, widespread use of penicillin on the evolution of penicillin-resistant bacteria. More difficult to incorporate are perceptions of the effects of the use of pesticides, defoliants, artificial animal-growth stimulants, and similar products on human populations, through the food-chain or the more immediate environment. Proposals for the use of such products are not part of human-project research, although use affects human populations in ways that cannot always be foreseen. The CIOMS Guidelines can have more influence over the effects of human biomedical research on the environment than over the effects of environmental research on human beings.

Developments in perception

Since the 1982 Guidelines were prepared, a number of developments have occurred in perceptions of biomedical research involving human subjects. Some of these refine issues addressed in the Guidelines, several add dimensions, and some apply in opposition to the thrust of the 1982 document. It has been seen above, for instance, that the Guidelines are applicable not only to research subjects but also to socially-structured population groups and to collections of individuals who have no personal interactions but who meet the recruitment criteria of studies. Questions must therefore be addressed of these collectivities' consent, confidentiality, protection from harm and entitlements to benefit from studies.

An esoteric and indirect development has been some recognition that the 1982 Guidelines were unfortunately titled. They were called "Proposed International Guidelines," meaning that they were put forward or propounded by CIOMS. Some readers concluded, however, that their status was that of an agency's proposal that is submitted to a higher authority for consideration in order to be adopted. Accordingly, the document has been considered to have a contingent or incomplete status, and to await higher endorsement before taking effect. It cannot be determined whether the title reduced the authority or influence of the 1982 Guidelines. It is intended, however, that the revised version will bear a more direct title.

A number of areas are identified below in which perceptions have developed that are reflected in the process to revise the 1982 Guidelines.

Informed consent. Respect for subjects' adequately informed consent to participate in biomedical research remains of the greatest significance to both individual and group studies. It is recognized, however, that consent once given is not necessarily enduring. Subjects' consent has to be monitored in studies of any duration, since the quality of consensuality with which they begin may diminish in time, or become changed through forgetfulness or evolving perceptions of their purposes, features or implications. Investigators may therefore be asked how they intend to monitor subjects' continuing informed consent, accommodate the fading or withdrawal of consent, and keep subjects' relevant information up to date. For instance, if newly published research data answer questions that a long-term study was designed to address, its value may be reduced and its risk-to-benefit ratio will be affected; investigators may be required to show that they intend to deal with such an eventuality appropriately.

Free consent. Voluntariness similarly remains central to participation in individual and group studies. From their origins in the Nuremberg Code, guidelines have emphasized non-coercion, but attention has come to be given in addition to concerns about over-inducement of participation. Financial payment raises most obvious concern, particularly when high enough to induce subjects to accept risks that they otherwise would reject. Non-pecuniary inducements include access to otherwise unavailable medical care, for subjects or for their family members. Caution must be exercised lest investigators benefit unduly from or exploit subjects' deprivation of care or their poverty. As against this, however, subjects' participation may be suitably reciprocated. Sensitivity to local culture and legitimate expectations must be exercised to distinguish between improper inducement of consent and acceptable or required courteous reciprocity of collaboration.

Community-based research. It has been seen repeatedly above that revision of the 1982 Guidelines will be influenced by the 1991 guidelines for epidemiological studies. Communities that exist as social realities, composed of interacting individuals who identify themselves with one another, may be approached through their authentic leadership, which can speak credibly on members' behalf. Leaders cannot compel individual community members to do what the individuals oppose, but they may express consensuality for the community. In contrast, no such person may speak on behalf of a group of subjects that exists only as a statistical construct, composed of individuals joined only by their conformity to a scientific description in a research protocol of the types of subject intended to be recruited. For the purposes of the research, such individuals are not members of communities.

Pregnant and nursing women. A development has occurred that amounts almost to a reversal of the priorities that shaped the 1982 Guidelines. Until recently, the requirement of preventing risks in research caused investigators to exclude women who were or might be pregnant, or who were of child-bearing age, from drug and similar studies. It was feared that fetuses might be harmed, or that uncontrollable variables would be introduced to data by recruitment of subjects at different stages of pregnancy or of their menstrual cycles. The result has been the marketing of drugs and vaccines that have not been tested on women, for instance for effective dosage levels and for safety. These have sometimes caused women and fetuses to suffer harms that research could have prevented or minimized. It has become an ethical expectation of drug, vaccine and comparable studies that they be tested on the full range of the population for which they are proposed to be developed, including adult women. Proven or specifically suspected risk of harm to fetuses, such as mutagenicity or teratogenicity, will justify exclusion of pregnant women. Pregnant or nursing women are similarly usually unsuitable for clinical studies in which women who are not pregnant or nursing would be equally suitable. Generally, however, the practice of exclusion of women,

17

which was common up to 1982, has become a general rule of inclusion and of investigators having to explain exclusion.

Confidentiality. Perceptions regarding research subjects' confidentiality have evolved not so much in point of principle as in practice, affected by technological advances in the management of mass data. More data can now be electronically collected and linked, so that an individual's personal identifier can be used to collate and interpret information from many different sources. A comprehensive picture of the person's health, medical prescriptions, activities, purchases, diet, interests, domestic environment and, for instance, religious and political convictions, can be composed. Health data can be electronically researched more fully and accurately than by a research subject giving a medical history from recollection, and be amplified by similar data regarding a subject's family members. Such information may considerably assist genetic and other studies, but access to it may be a breach of confidentiality when identified individuals have not given their prior consent. The collection and electronic storage of research data may similarly be invaded in breach of subjects' confidentiality. As against this, however, the mass collection of data in electronic banks may allow aggregated data to be extracted without exposure of individually identifiable files, thus enhancing confidentiality. The revised Guidelines will recognize the potential of electronic data management.

Externally sponsored research. The 1982 Guidelines were drawn up with particular concern about their applicability to research conducted in developing countries, but they warrant further consideration of how they address research that is sponsored and funded externally to the host country. When principal investigators come from another country and act for that country or an international agency, cultural incompatibilities, misunderstandings or insensitivities may affect the conduct of the research or the interpretation of its findings. Comparable issues arise when the external sponsor is a commercial enterprise that promotes marketable products and funds its research without submitting protocols to external agencies for ethical review.

Ethical problems become most acute when a host country and the investigator's country do not share the same application or prioritization of ethical values. Cultural relativity and respect for international pluralism may conflict with ethical absolutism in defence of basic or threshold values; fears of ethical imperialism may conflict with fears of compromise of minimum ground-rules of research ethics. How and whether consent is to be sought from prospective subjects who are not accustomed to exercising self-determination, and whether introducing the concept of individual autonomy will improperly and irreversibly change a community based on customary authority or patriarchy, are issues that revision of the 1982 Guidelines will have to address.

Compensation for injury. It seems a matter of simple justice that a subject accidentally injured by participation in a study should receive compensation. Legally, however, this may not be self-evident, since a subject who is adequately informed of the risk and freely agrees to take it may be said in law to have assumed the risk. Informing a subject that injury may occur through no fault of the investigator, sponsor or other agent may legally transfer responsibility for the injury to the person who freely and knowingly takes the risk. Ethically, however, this may be inadequate. The investigator or sponsor has more awareness of the extent and nature of risks to subjects, and is almost invariably in a better position to provide redress. An agent who is at fault should bear liability to compensate an innocent victim, but even when injury occurs through no fault of an investigator, sponsor or other proponent of a study, an injured subject should be entitled to compensation. This may be a money payment or medical care that maximizes relief or both. The revision of the 1982 Guidelines will take into account the need to protect subjects beyond the taking of due precautions against future injury.

Generally unchanged areas. Ethical priorities and issues have not changed since 1982 in several important areas of biomedical research. The involvement in studies of such vulnerable subjects as children and mentally impaired people remains liable to critical scrutiny, and governed by such principles as that they should not be recruited when adult and unimpaired subjects would serve the purposes of studies equally well. Opinions have evolved to some extent on the recruitment of prison populations in studies in which non-prison populations would be equally suitable. Prisoners' liability to coercion and their severely restricted self-determination cast doubt on their capacity to decide to enter studies that prison administrations have accommodated within institutions, or will allow prisoners to serve outside prison grounds. As opposed to this, however, prisoners may claim that participation in studies need not involve risks of escape, smuggling or other violations of prison rules, and represents one of their few opportunities for altruism, rehabilitation and restoration of self-esteem. The debate has not produced any new perceptions that would seem to compel fundamental rethinking of the approach taken in 1982. The same is true of studies that recruit members of disciplined services such as the military or the police, or employees of hospitals or research laboratories in which the studies are conducted.

Developments not ready for guidelines

Some research occurring in biomedicine today is either exciting or alarming, depending on one's viewpoint. This research will be considered in the revision of the 1982 Guidelines, but the issues and responses to them may be too uncertain or unsettled to be made objects of specific ethical guidance. The 1992 Guidelines may have a general applicability, as indeed may other codes of research-ethics.

Embryo and fetal research has become liable to quite strict control in some developed countries, under specific codes of practice regarding such research itself or under guidelines on treatment of infertility. The moral status that unborn human life is considered to possess affects what types of research are considered appropriate. There is no international consensus on these matters. Similarly, research that uses tissues from aborted fetuses, for instance fetal brain cells, for implantation into patients with Parkinson's disease, is contentious, and not the object of ethical agreement. It may be considered inappropriate to propose principles to guide research practices that individuals, medical organizations and governments may consider should not be permitted at all. Research may proceed ethically if it is dissociated from a woman's decision on abortion, and if her well-being is not compromised in arranging the timing and technique of the procedure. It may be premature, however, to propose guidelines.

Genetic research in the form of so-called genetic-engineering studies tends to have a therapeutic purpose for those to whom it is offered, and in any event may be unobjectionable, according to the 1982 Guidelines, when the effects are limited to individual patients. In contrast to such somatic-cell treatment, germ-line treatment changes the genetic character of the treated patient's children, and of each successive generation. Preventing the genetic transmission of harmful conditions and predispositions may be benign, but a margin of unpredictability exists in such work that will affect future generations. There are limits to how far parents can consent to research that will affect their children. Moreover, parents may have a conflict of interest when research or treatment designed to benefit them may affect their subsequently conceived children. Results of the Human Genome Project are likely to give a better understanding of genetic transmission, which may furnish a more reliable base for ethical guidelines than currently exists.

As the proportion of elderly people rises in many countries, particularly in the developed world, geriatric research is increasing. Much of it concerns the physical and neurological effects of aging, but studies into the living conditions of elderly people, particularly those suffering from age-related disorders, are also expanding. Although elderly people are distinguishable in medical terms from people in their middle years of life, much as infants, children and adolescents are distinguishable, research proposed for the elderly may be appropriately covered by sensitive application of the 1982 Guidelines. It may be objectionable or dysfunctional to separate a category of elderly adults and stereotype them as physically or cognitively disabled. The field of geriatric research remains open to development, but it is not obvious that the present revision of the 1982 Guidelines should attempt further refinement of principles in this regard.

Ethical review procedures

The aim of the 1982 Guidelines to encourage and facilitate establishment of prospective ethical review committees has been at best only partially achieved. Particularly but not only in developing countries, such review does not occur or does not conform to reasonably rigorous standards of independent scrutiny. The revision of the existing Guidelines will be futile if the version that results will not be applied to many of the studies to which the new guidelines will be relevant.

It is recognized that in some circumstances, particularly in developing countries, potential committee-members of appropriate expertise are not conveniently accessible. The problem concerns scientific peer-review of proposals as well as ethical review but, since it is a condition of ethical approval of studies that they be shown to be scientifically sound, concerns over scientific and ethical review interact.

The 1982 Guidelines on ethical review procedures may fall short of the ideal more in practice than in principle. Since 1982 the process of review has become better understood and the literature on the subject has expanded, with the result that much more is now perceived that will contribute to fine-tuning of the 1982 principles. CIOMS is aware of the role that international agencies, including itself, may perform in providing scientific and other personnel to assist ethical review in countries where convenient access to such personnel is difficult. Efforts to make guidelines effective are administrative rather than normative, and do not have to be written into the guidelines themselves. Accordingly, the revised version of the 1982 Guidelines regarding ethical review procedures may refine the original text in light of subsequent experience, and leave it to other documents and dynamics to address what CIOMS and others recognize must be done to make the Guidelines universally effective.

INFORMED CONSENT

INDIVIDUAL CONSENT:
A PERSPECTIVE OF DEVELOPING COUNTRIES

B.O. Osuntokun*

Research in human subjects is done and has to be done in all countries, developed and developing. As pointed out in 1982, "consideration is thus required in developed and developing countries alike as to whether prevailing legal provisions and administrative arrangements ensure that human rights and welfare of subjects involved in biomedical research are adequately considered and protected in conformity with the ethical principles prescribed in the World Medical Association's Declaration of Helsinki"[1].

Ideally, all biomedical research involving human subjects should be conducted in compliance with the three ethical principles: respect for persons, beneficence and distributive justice. Respect for persons underscores two fundamental ethical issues: autonomy, and protection of those with diminished autonomy. Autonomous individuals are those who are capable of making decisions about themselves and acting on those decisions, and they should be treated with respect for their capacity for self-determination. They have the option to choose whether or not to participate in a research project. Research involving human subjects should be conducted only with the informed consent of the subjects. Those whose autonomy is diminished or who are vulnerable in other ways may be unable to protect their interests to the same extent and level that autonomous people can. Such vulnerable individuals should be given additional protection to ensure their well-being and protect their rights when they are asked to participate in research involving human subjects.

Valid consent involves three elements.[2] First an individual or group or community must be competent to understand and assess information about the research and make an informed choice. Second, consent must be voluntary. The decision of a prospective subject or group or community should not be biased by improper influences. A poor person may not have the option to decline to participate in research offering monetary compensation. Third, the prospective subject or group or community must be given the detailed truthful information necessary to make a considered judgement about whether to participate.

In my assessment of recent views on ethical issues in biomedical research involving human subjects, respect for persons and informed consent have received the greatest attention (often controversial). Many of these views have been motivated by proposals to carry out trials of human-immunodeficiency-virus (HIV) vaccine in developing countries.

---

* Professor of Medicine (Neurology), University of Ibadan, Ibadan, Nigeria.

One eminent participant at a conference on the topic held in October 1991 is quoted as saying "How can we create one set of rules that will work for Buddhists in Thailand, Moslems in Africa and Christians in Brazil?" The anonymous commentator who reported the above went on: "For example in many African countries, there is no concept of the individual beyond one's role in the community. Who will consent for subjects in such culture? ... in some tribes a woman's sexual activity is dictated by her mother-in-law. The subjugation of women by their husbands is common throughout Africa".[3] These outworn and largely anachronistic views could apply, if at all, to small isolated communities in a continent, where people, when allowed, can freely cast votes to choose their political leaders. Besides, the existence of the concept of autonomy where individuals perceive themselves as part of a collective is not confined to some primitive isolated African tribal communities, but can be found in some religious sects in the Western world.

The CIOMS Proposed Guidelines of 1982, the revision of which is the theme of this Conference, deal extensively with the ethical principle of informed consent. Similarly, informed consent of individuals and communities is extensively dealt with in International Guidelines for Ethical Review of Epidemiological Studies, developed by CIOMS, WHO and the International Epidemiological Association during 1990 and 1991.[4] Judging from respondents to a survey of the CIOMS 1982 Guidelines, the areas that require amplification and review appear to be ethical issues associated with large-scale trials of vaccines and drugs, transnational research, and experimentation involving members of vulnerable population groups. Such review would take into consideration conceptual developments that have taken place since 1982 in fundamental ethical principles and their application; and new proposals and recommendations such as the United Nations draft Convention for the Prevention and Suppression of Unlawful Human Experimentation. In addition, progress in scientific knowledge and research techniques, together with increased awareness of differing circumstances of potential research subjects, pose new challenges to the application of the CIOMS 1982 Guidelines in specific settings.

My task is to consider the needs for review from the perspective of developing countries, the consent of individuals and agreement of communities to participation in research, including concepts of disclosure and consent, inducements to consent, selection of subjects, special concerns of disadvantaged or vulnerable populations, and problems of fully informing and gaining the agreement of communities. So as to avoid repetition of previously published or expressed views by CIOMS and the International Guidelines for Ethical Review of Epidemiological Studies,[1,3-5] I would indicate my concurrence without quoting them.

Ethical universalism, pluralism, dictatorship and imperialism

One basic topical issue is whether the fundamental ethical principles, particularly those that embody autonomy, should be universally applicable. Are ethical standards for research involving human subjects relative, to be weighed against cultural values and modified accordingly, or are they, like scientific standards, absolute? Are ethical principles to be regarded as table manners, whose nature is irrelevant as long as they are indigenous? It has been pointed out that informed consent holds a central place in the ethical justification of research involving human subjects and that it is the first-stated and longest principle of the Nuremberg Code.[6]

> "The voluntary consent of the human subject is absolutely essential. This means that the person involved should have the legal capacity to give consent, should be so situated as to be able to exercise free power of choice, without intervention of any element of force, fraud, duress, overreaching or other ulterior form of constraint or coercion; and should have sufficient knowledge and comprehension of the elements of the subject matter involved so as to enable him to make an understanding and enlightened decision. This latter element requires that before the acceptance of an affirmative decision by the experimental subject, there should be made known to him, the nature, duration and purpose of the experiment, the method and means by which it is to be conducted; all inconveniences and hazards reasonably to be expected; and the effects upon his health or person which may possibly come from his participation in the experiment."

The fundamental attributes of valid consent are that consent must be voluntary, "legally competent", "informed", and "comprehending". Could these attributes change from place to place, from one culture to another, etc. or could they, like fundamental human rights, have the status of ethical rules or norms. There are well-known side-effects of informed consent, undesirable to the subjects (e.g. anxiety, and other psychosomatic effects) and to the outcome of the experiment,[7] but no one has convincingly argued that informed consent should be abandoned in Western societies.

Some eminent ethicists believe that the informed-consent standards of the Declaration of Helsinki are not universally valid[6,8] and those who hold such views have been described as ethical pluralists. Others believe that all research, wherever it is conducted, should be justified according to universally applicable standards[9], and they have been labelled ethical universalists, who want to impose ethical imperialism or dictatorship on others, particularly in the developing countries. I subscribe to the middle-of-the-road view that there must be certain well-defined ethical minimal standards, respected by all, below which no one must fall and which can change only a little from place to place. Angell[9] reflects this view incisively: "There must be a core of human rights that we would wish to see honoured universally, despite local variations in their superficial aspects... The force of local custom or law cannot justify abuses of certain fundamental rights and the right of self-determination on which the doctrine of informed consent is based is one of them." It is relevant to state that Levine,[6] perhaps the leading pluralist, admits that some ethical universalism is desirable: "the conduct of research involving human subjects must not violate any universally applicable ethical standards... and there are limits to how much cultural relativism ought to be tolerated... The principle of respect for persons is one of the universally accepted applicable ethical standards". He went on to express some reservation that respect for persons is universally applicable when stated at the level of formality employed by Immanuel Kant: "so act as to treat humanity, whether in thine own person or in that of any other, in every case as an end withal, never as a means only."

We must remember that the Nuremberg Code came into being less than five decades ago and that most of the ethical norms and regulations now in place in Western countries emerged from a time of outright scandal and abuse in medical research, of which Nuremberg and Tuskegee are the paradigmatic watchwords.[10] It was only in 1974 that the United States Congress established the National Commission for the Protection of Human Subjects of Biomedical and Behavioural Research, asking it to "conduct a comprehensive investigation and study to identify the basic ethical principles which should underlie the conduct of biomedical and behavioral research involving human subjects..." In the United Kingdom in the 1960s the incisive documentation of unethical practice, based on published papers in scientific journals, revolutionized the views about ethical norms in research in the United States in which human rights were flagrantly disregarded.[11] The principles of bioethics have undergone fundamental changes in Western societies in the last five decades. The truth is that in many Third World countries bioethics is emerging only slowly (if at all) as a concept, but this does not make it right that good rules and standards should not be learned, accepted and adopted in such countries. People and communities can change, and they do change, and in ethical terms developing countries do not need to reinvent the wheel. For example, as a neurologist, I found that the great reluctance of African patients to giving a history constituted enormous difficulty in neurological practice. They expected the Western-trained doctor to discover symptoms, just as the Babalawo or the diviner (native doctor) usually did (and still does).[12] In my experience, and within three decades, that attitude has changed completely and patients now give a history.

Informed consent and related issues: perception in the context of developing countries.

As stated earlier, I subscribe to the guidelines and views expressed in the CIOMS *International Guidelines for Ethical Review of Epidemiological Studies*,[4] and the basic ethical principles in the CIOMS (1982) *Proposed International Guidelines for Biomedical Research Involving Human Subjects*.[1] The following represents my emphasis.

The cornerstones of the ethics of biomedical research involving human subjects are informed meaningful consent of each subject and a proper procedure for obtaining the consent, approved on ethical grounds by a suitably qualified body independent of the investigators. Where for ethically approved research it is impossible to obtain individual informed consent, vicarious consent should be obtained from parents in the case of children or from a legal guardian, as in the case of the mentally retarded or incapacitated. The subjects must retain autonomy and be free to withdraw without incurring any penalty as to the right to access to health services and without infringement of the doctor-patient relationship. The subjects must not be exposed to any unreasonable risk. Mechanisms for assessing risk and compensating for accidents must be built into the research procedure, as specified in the 1982 CIOMS Guidelines.[1] The interests of the subjects must always prevail over the interests of science and society, as specified by the Declaration of Helsinki.

In certain cultures the rule on autonomy of a mentally competent adult may be modified. In some parts of Africa, the consent of a husband has to be obtained before a wife can be expected to give consent. In my own opinion, even then the husband's consent should not be a substitute for that of the wife, but rather an additional consent, and it should not override the wife's refusal.

Some have argued that in some developing countries it would be valid to obtain vicarious consent by community leaders for research involving entire communities or large segments of them, and that, in certain circumstances, once this was done, informed consent from individuals would not be necessary. I do not agree with this view. The assertion that in some central African cultures the concept of personhood differs fundamentally from that in Western culture, that "person" as an individual does not exist in the local language of some Bantus, and that "personhood" is defined by one's tribe, village or social group[8] can be true only in respect of some small ethnic groups: it is not true of most parts of Black Africa.

In my opinion and that of many others, consent by community leaders could complement informed consent of individuals or facilitate obtaining informed consent of prospective subjects, as long as the research procedure involves direct contact with individuals. There are instances, however, when the rights of individuals may be subservient to that of the community, if incidental infringement of individual liberties is decisively outweighed by the benefit to the community as a whole. Examples include research in, or measures involving, modification of the environment (vector control) and research on public health measures (new prophylactic or immunizing agents), new treatment of water supply, or nutritional supplements to staple foods. In such instances the ultimate decision to undertake the research would rest with the responsible public health authority.[1] Even then "all possible means should be used to inform the community concerned of the aims of the research, the advantages expected from it, and any possible hazards or inconveniences. If feasible, dissenting individuals should have the option of withholding their participation. Whatever the circumstances, the ethical considerations and safeguards applied to research on individuals must be translated, in every possible respect, into the community context".[1]

In epidemiological research it is ethically important, especially in developing countries, where health care services may be grossly inadequate, that facilities be provided to deal with acute medical conditions and incidental illnesses. It is also important that, when necessary, the researchers should take appropriate steps to inform the community of the results. In one country endemic for yellow fever, in 1985, researchers found serological evidence of low community-immunity and published the result in a good scientific journal. Neither the researchers nor the public-health authorities (who were not aware of the results of the research) did anything, and a year later a virulent epidemic of yellow fever broke out.

For international cooperation and national research needs in developing countries, researchers from developed countries often carry out research on human beings in developing countries. Ideally such collaborative research, usually sponsored by external agencies, including international organizations, or by nationally-based funding agencies such as foundations, research councils, universities and research-based pharmaceutical companies, involves researchers who are citizens of the developing countries where the research is being done. This is to ensure that some technology transfer or building of local problem-solving capacity takes place. It is unethical to carry out what has been referred to as "parachute" or "helicopter" research projects, in which researchers from developed countries go to developing countries, carry out and complete a research project with little or no involvement of researchers from the developing countries, and then leave. In some instances results of such research projects had been published even before data were shared with the developing countries where the work was done. The externally sponsored research project must be approved by the national or local ethical committee in the country where the research is being done and also by an appropriate ethical committee of the developed country or countries from which the researchers come. It is a correct ethical principle that the externally sponsored research should serve local or national rather than external interests.

Not infrequently in the recent past, especially in countries with no adequate mechanism for management of research, and hence no national or institutional regulations on ethics of research involving human subjects, researchers from developed countries carried out research without apparently complying with ethical guidelines that would have been appropriate or required in their own countries. I believe that there should be some minimal universal ethical standards that should apply to research involving human subjects anywhere in the world: those already specified or about to be specified by CIOMS and WHO[1,4,5] are adequate for this purpose. Where developing countries in which externally sponsored research is to be carried out do not have national or institutional regulations, those of the developed countries and their institutions that are sponsoring the research should apply. Cultural modifications such as the additional consent of husband or community leaders should supplement, not substitute for, the accepted ethical norm of informed consent of individuals. The minimal ethical standards, e.g. those of CIOMS, should be regarded as absolute, like scientific standards. For in biomedical ethics of research involving human beings, as in science, and not as in politics, there should be no compromise to allow the force of local custom or law to justify abuses of certain fundamental rights, such as the right of self-determination, on which the doctrine of informed consent is based. When researchers from developed countries compromise the basic ethical principles in research involving human subjects in developing countries, they invite the justifiable accusation of ethical imperialism[9,13] or exploitation or dictatorship. They should not carry out in a developing country research involving human subjects that could be done in a developed country. For example, it has been suggested that, because human immunodeficiency virus (HIV) infection is common in certain parts of Africa, testing of low-cost HIV candidate vaccines should be carried out mainly in that continent.[13,14] This would be unethical. Both the developed and the developing countries must make sure that such unethical practice does not occur.

The other side of the coin is when clinical trials of drugs are carried out in developed countries and the results are then "extrapolated" to developing countries; this could be unethical. It is now well established that there are variations in the pharmacokinetics and pharmacodynamics of drugs, and of drug toxicity, in relation to diet, lifestyle, racially and genetically determined metabolic differences, and balanced genetic polymorphisms. An example of the last is glucose-6-phosphate-dehydrogenase deficiency, which increases the susceptibility of Black Africans to massive haemolysis in reaction to such drugs as the 4-amino quinolines (primaquine and pamaquine, used for radical cure of malaria). Chinese, Black Africans and Afro-Americans and Caucasians differ in the pharmacokinetics and pharmacodynamics of beta blockers. Chinese have shown a much larger reduction in heart rate and blood pressure, and also metabolized propranolol more efficiently, than American whites.[15] The reduction of blood pressure by propranolol was less in Black Americans than in white subjects.[16] The differences could be partly explained by the variation in the genetically variable member of the cytochrome P-450 system known as debrisoquine hydroxylase. It is well recognized that there are racial differences in other drug-metabolizing enzymes in humans, such as alcohol dehydrogenase and acetylating enzyme for isonicotinic acid anhydride. Ideally the multinational drug-companies should carry out separate clinical trials of new drugs in major countries and major racial groups. Such differential testing would place unending and unnecessary burdens on both suppliers and consumers of drugs, and hence it has been suggested that an international organization such as WHO should provide guiding principles.[17] It is, however, crystal clear on the evidence available that it is ethically important to assess drug efficacy and effectiveness in different populations in order to detect differences in racial and ethnic groups, and that the results of studies performed on one population are not necessarily applicable to other populations. It is no longer valid to confine well-controlled pre-marketing studies of drugs to groups of patients in Western countries.

A basic principle in therapeutic trials, which is related to the issue of racial and ethnic differences in drug efficacy and effectiveness, is the concept of exclusion criteria. It is debatable whether it is ethically justifiable to exclude certain patients (on the basis of age, severity of disease, co-existing disease, difficulty in enrolling) from controlled trials and to apply or extrapolate the results to all groups in day-to-day practices, including those groups who have been excluded from the trials.[18,19]

It has also been suggested that, just as informed consent is necessary for a subject to be enrolled in a research project such as a controlled drug-trial, similar informed consent should be obtained before a subject is excluded from a therapeutic trial that may be beneficial to the subject.[18] "Parallel tracks" are now being created for patients outside drug trials to enable them to receive unapproved drugs, because of patients' unwillingness to agree to be randomized, and of protocol restriction when it is unknown whether the drug will be more helpful than harmful. This is unethical. What is being suggested is that all available patients who might benefit should be included in a randomized trail.

When research and controlled trials carried out in developing countries have proved a treatment efficacious and effective, it is ethically desirable that the new treatment should remain available and affordable to the population. It is understandable that market forces are involved in pricing new drugs. An ideal situation is that typified by the availability of ivermectin for mass treatment of filariasis, although special considerations made it possible for the manufacturer to make the drug available free of charge. The opposite is the highly prohibitive cost of eflornithine (dimethylfluoroornithine), the only new drug in three decades to prove efficacious in the treatment of African trypanosomiasis, but at a cost of over US$ 280 for a course of treatment.

Some general conclusions

Biomedical ethical issues, guidelines, principles and regulations cut across national boundaries and often have universal implications. Though peoples and cultures differ, certain values are common to all. In this context, the most important is respect for human dignity, and this should not be negotiable. In many developing countries there is no mechanism for management of research. For example, only 22 of 45 countries in Black Africa have medical research councils or their equivalents, and only few of those have national ethical committees or their equivalents. In developing countries, institutional ethical committees in medical schools and in research institutes are often ineffective. Many developing countries have no equivalents of the USA Food and Drug Administration System or institutional review boards and the control they exercise. However, most have professional statutory regulatory bodies and these perform some functions as ethical watchdogs for professional ethical behaviour. It is important that every country should have a dynamic mechanism for dealing with ethical problems as well as for regulating ethical norms in medical practice and research. Such a mechanism must be responsive to changes within and outside the country, and must take into consideration the views of the majority of the citizens.[20] It may involve the establishment of a national medical ethics commission, and regional, local and institutional ethics committees. The national medical ethics committee would be responsible for formulating national policies on ethics in medical practice and research, and must also evaluate for approval all research projects that are externally funded or sponsored: it should have access to lawmakers and the highest policy-makers of the ministry of health.

Ethical guidelines should be dynamic, and periodically reviewed. Ethical principles should be more like statutes, difficult to change. It should also be realized that communities do change, become "deculturated" and acculturated. Obedience to tribal leaders[21] has disappeared in some communities within a generation. In many developing countries, political emancipation and periodic exposure to vote-seeking harangues have changed perceptions of collective leadership and of the role of the individual in the society and community. People are increasingly becoming better educated and more amenable to change. They change cultural habits. Human rights should be inviolable, but they are meant to be used to serve the society, and when they cease to do so, or are used to threaten the society, society has the right to protect itself. The researcher, whose duty is to seek knowledge, must first comply with basic ethical principles that regulate research involving human subjects. The main thrust of biomedical ethics in health-care and research is to preserve human dignity and social justice and the good reputation of the researchers.

For many developing countries leap-frogging centuries in development and undergoing epidemiological transition, conflicts not infrequently occur in the constant flux of life and raise ethical problems, particularly against a background of rapid change in Western medical and technological knowledge. Resolution is not impossible, once the necessary legal, administrative, political and health care mechanisms are established. For example, traditional medicine does not need to be abolished, but it should be evaluated, and strictly it would be unethical not to do so if a majority of a community continues to use the services.

I should like to end on a personal note. In the last decade since the CIOMS guidelines were proposed, I have been involved with colleagues in several research projects involving human subjects, in Nigerian communities and in such a non-Westernized community as the Cree Indians of Northern Manitoba. We have had no difficulty in complying with the CIOMS Proposed Guidelines. Perhaps the revised ethical guidelines should address more cogently than before the duties and obligations of the researchers and the sanctions applicable, as well as the rights and wrongs as they apply to research subjects.

References

1. *Proposed International Guidelines for Biomedical Research Involving Human Subjects.* Geneva, CIOMS, 1982, p. 4.
2. National Commission for the Protection of Human Subjects of Biomedical and Behavioural Research. *The Belmont Report: Ethical Principles and Guidelines for the Protection of Human Subjects of Research.* Washington, DC, US Dept. of Health, Education and Welfare. Publication (OS), 78-0013, 1979.
3. Trials of HIV vaccine planned for developing countries. *Brit. Med. J,* 1991, 303: 1219-20.
4. *International guidelines for ethical review of epidemiological studies.* Geneva, CIOMS, 1991.
5. Levine, RJ. Vaccine and drug trials — ethical issues. In: Z. Bankowski, J.H. Bryant & J.M.Last (eds.), *Ethics and epidemiology: international guidelines.* Geneva, Council for International Organizations of Medical Sciences, 1991.
6. Levine, RJ. Informed consent: some challenges to the universal validity of the Western model. In: Z. Bankowski, [as in reference 5].
7. Marsh, BT. Informed consent, — help or hindrance. *J. Roy, Soc. Med.* 1990, 83: 603-5.
8. DeCraemer, W. A Cross-cultural perspective on personhood. *Milbank Memorial Fund Quarterly,* 1983, 61: 19-34.
9. Angell, M. Ethical imperialism? Ethics in international collaborative clinical research. *N. Engl. J. Med.,* 1988, 319: 1081-3.

10. Caplan, AL. Ethics and clinical research. *Lancet*, 1990, 336: 1261.
11. Beecher, HK. Ethics and clinical research. *N. Engl. J. Med.*, 1966, 274: 1354-60.
12. Osuntokun, B.O., Neurological disorders in Nigeria. In: Spillane, J.D. *Tropical Neurology*, London, Oxford University Press, 1973. p. 162.
13. Barry, M. Ethical considerations of human investigations in developing countries. The AIDS dilemma. *N. Engl. J. Med.*, 1988, 319: 1083-5.
14. Christakis, N.A. The ethical design of an AIDS vaccine trial in Africa. *Hastings Cent. Rep.* 1988, 18: 31-7.
15. Zhou, H.H., Koshakji, R.P., Silberstein, D.J., Wilkinson, G.P., Wood, A.J.J. Racial differences in drug response: altered sensitivity to and clearance of propranolol in men of Chinese descent as compared with American whites. *N. Engl. J. Med.*, 1989, 320: 565-570.
16. Freis, E.D. Antihypertensive agents. In: Kalow, W., Guedde, H.W. and Agarwal, P. (eds) *Ethnic differences in reactions to drugs and xenobiotics.* p. 312-322. New York, Alan Liss, 1986.
17. Kalow, W. Race and therapeutic drug response. *N. Engl. J. Med.*, 1989, 320: 588-9.
18. Chalmers, T.C. Ethical implications of rejecting patients for clinical trials. *JAMA*, 1990, 263: 865.
19. Greenfield, S. The state of outcome research. Are we on target? *N. Engl. J. Med.*, 1989, 320: 1142-3.
20. Davies, N.E., Felder, L.H. Applying brakes to the runaway American Health Care System. *JAMA*, 1990, 263: 73-6.
21. Ajayi, O.O. Taboos and clinical research in West Africa. *J. Med. Ethics*, 1980, 6: 61-3.

INFORMED CONSENT: PROTECTING THE VULNERABLE

C. de Sweemer-Ba*

Introduction

Reflecting on my subject I have felt the same fascination and dissatisfaction as I feel when trying to interpret a Rorschach test. The "vulnerable": who are they? Against whom or what are ethical committees or researchers protecting them?

Two years ago CIOMS called a conference on ethics and epidemiology, which resulted in *International guidelines for ethical review of epidemiological studies*[1] and in published proceedings.[2] Both show great concern for vulnerable individuals and populations. Most of what is said seems directly applicable as ethical guidelines for any population-based study or any research on vulnerable human subjects. This paper summarizes and reaffirms the "epidemiological guidelines", and stresses the need to deepen out the reflection and perhaps refocus the issue.

There is cause for dissatisfaction at the state of the art of protecting the vulnerable, both in health education and disease control and in research. There has been much progress from an individualistic medical deontology to an understanding that both macro- and micro-ethical principles need to be applied and that both individual and community rights need to be recognized. However, we seem to accommodate ourselves to fundamental contradictions: the researcher (or, worse, the ethical committees) as the lone Don Quixote defending the rights of the "vulnerable", who day and night are made more vulnerable by society at large. Our weapons seem strangely inadequate — largely ritualized normative procedures, which are supposed to result from consequentialist and thus contextual ethics. Many of us seem quite pleased: television journalism and many sociological and anthropological research studies have cultivated in us an ability to feel better by their simply condemning causes of human misery and inequity, while distancing us from the people concerned.

My consolation is that at least some of us are not at ease with our present approach and that, increasingly, people, "human subjects", question our right to make ethical or other decisions for them. To live by consequential and contextual ethics means that one knows or tries to predict consequences, and that one has a basic knowledge of the context that one seeks to extend. In fact, the context will be a major factor in determining the nature, severity, and timing of consequences. Our knowledge of both context and consequences is never complete, and one needs to accept a degree of uncertainty about them at the

---

* International Development Research Centre, Dakar, Senegal.

onset of research, but they should be of continuing concern to an ethical researcher before, during and after the research. Especially before the research, both researcher and ethical committee should use literature review and qualitative anthropological approaches to learn more about the context and the likely consequences.

Wherever possible — and exceptions should be rare — prospective subjects of research should be involved through focus-group or other group dynamics in giving their views of the context and likely consequences as well as of how to maximize beneficence and minimize harm. Let people speak: they have a voice, they should be heard. In the 1980s gay activists taught us so. In developing countries dissatisfaction at not being consulted has been brewing among the people since colonial times. It found early organized expression in Nigeria during the 1930s. Ola Rotimi reflects it in his historical masterpiece, *Hopes of the Living Dead*: a group of leprosy patients who underwent early clinical testing of DDS organize themselves when the experiment is prematurely interrupted because of the departure of the researcher; they seek a voice in regard to treatment, livelihood and solidarity, and become a true healing community. But it should hardly take the failure of a researcher before this can happen.

One of the enormous benefits of participation of the vulnerable in understanding context and likely consequences is that they speak from life experience, with all the forces that impinge upon them, including fear and self-censure. The researcher thus is educated and introduced into people's unique worlds, and in turn can start stimulating reflection on viable opportunities for defence or change. It is also remarkable that epidemiologists have, with military precision, studied high-risk groups, which can then be targeted, but that very few epidemiologists or social scientists have studied the sociology and anthropology of vulnerability.

The vulnerable

The list in the *International guidelines for ethical review of epidemiological studies*[1] may be divided into four categories:
1. Those who would be capable of informed consent but are not given the right to the necessary autonomy by their own society at large; examples are women, handicapped people, and prisoners.
2. Those who might be unduly influenced or tricked into consent unless very special precaution is taken to present simple and clear information: examples are members of communities unfamiliar with modern medical concepts.
3. Those who, under any circumstances, might not be capable of informed consent; examples are children, and many of the mentally ill.
4. Those dependent upon the researchers for their livelihood or studies; examples are medical students.

Once "vulnerability" has been broken down into these four categories it is clear that the first obligation on researchers or ethical review committees is to ask what groups of people have been rendered "vulnerable" by the particular society in which they plan to work. Those listed above are only a first indication and the list needs to be adapted to each society. Perhaps a checklist could be put at the disposal of researchers and committees, particularly for the first category of vulnerable, which is likely to be the most diverse, according to the social, cultural and political mores of a society.

In the first category it should be remembered that in all societies the recognized right to autonomy tends to vary by sex, age (too young, too old), social status, caste, ethnic origin, level of modern education; degree of perceived foreign origin, such as migrants, refugees, nomads, freed slaves; degree of economic participation, such as breadwinner or economic dependent, jobless or beggar. In many societies unmarried adults, sterile women or women with daughters only, and elderly with no living offspring are also particularly vulnerable, as are people with "shameful" or "supernatural" diseases (syphilis, tuberculosis, leprosy, leucoderma) or sensory loss or loss of limbs. Each society has its own variants and some societies are more unjust than others towards the vulnerable.

In the second category, each society, even outside the developing world, has groups or small clusters that are unfamiliar with modern medical concepts: usually the less educated, the poor, the old, the geographically isolated, the rural, the language minorities, or the occupationally despised (e.g., sex workers). It should be assumed that in the developing world the great majority of both the educated and the uneducated have had little exposure to modern medical concepts.

In the third category of those "incapable" of informed consent are included also the mentally retarded as well as people who are unconscious or dying.

However, there is a dangerous ambiguity in that the capacity for informed consent is not binary but rather varies by degrees, and can often be compensated for by patiently conducted group or individual discussion.

"Vulnerability" has a mixture of determinants, all of which connote that the humanity of members of "vulnerable" groups is diminished or even absent, and that therefore:

1. They cannot make decisions even for themselves;
2. They have no right to speak in public (*pas de voix dans le chapitre*);
3. They often have no right to demand even the fulfilment of their basic needs (food, water, medical care, etc.) and often have to scrape by on left-overs;
4. Any full community member can order them to work, reprimand them, punish them, chase them away, shut them up;

5. Societies tend to frown upon or even forbid the banding together or organizing of any of these groups except as work-teams or for entertainment or religious purposes; their leaders are in general not respected by society at large except in so far as they claim adherence to the dominant ethos;
6. Often, dangerous and exhausting work is reserved for them, exposing them to mechanical, chemical and infectious hazards;
7. They are often given reduced access to survival resources (food, clean water, health services, habitat and land, health information); therefore, once exposed to a hazard they have less defences.

Each society automatically invites and pressures even researchers to fall into a trap, increasing the powerlessness and vulnerability of vulnerable people.

How is this situation to be avoided? Still another set of normative ethical procedures will not do the trick; rather a humble return to experiment with a judicious mix of consequential, contextual meta-ethics and humanistic activism by the adventurous few with fire in the belly. Indeed, beneficence to vulnerable populations includes contributing towards making them conscious of their rights, towards their empowerment, and towards the awakening of their dormant faculties.

True progress depends on studying in each specific society who the "vulnerable" are and how society maintains and increases individual and group vulnerability. Such a study needs to be carried out in each society, because many of the determinants are economic, cultural and historical, and opportunities for corrective action are even more diverse.

As medical researchers can hardly be expected to be fully aware of the degree of vulnerability of every group with which they are likely to work, national ethical review committees might arrange that national studies be carried out to highlight this problem and determine the degree of vulnerability of the major groups and their structure.

Selection of vulnerable subjects for research

Once it is determined that certain groups or individuals are vulnerable, their selection as research subjects should take into account the following considerations:

— Does the disease under consideration occur uniquely or more frequently, or more severely, or with a different clinical evolution among the vulnerable (principle of equity and fit)?

— Is the experimental prevention or treatment likely if successful to be available to them in the near future at reasonable cost (beneficence)?

— Are the risks and burdens of participation excessive, given their fragile state (non-maleficence)?

Whenever the study is unlikely to improve the condition of the vulnerable by selecting them as study subjects, or the risks and burdens seem excessive for them, they should not be selected. This should not mean that all studies with vulnerable subjects are banned, but it should impose on all researchers who include them or select them preferentially the requirement to prove that their selection is necessary to improve the lot of the vulnerable and that the study will cause them no excessive risks or burdens.[3]

Particular attention needs to be drawn to the safety testing of vaccines. Safety tests should normally be undertaken first on individuals whose general state of health seems robust, and it is only when safety seems assured at least for the healthy, well nourished, non-vulnerable individual that it should be tried with at-risk individuals or groups, who, on the average, are more fragile. The vulnerable often cannot be distinguished from groups at risk of a great variety of nutritional deficiencies and infectious diseases. The same social, political and cultural factors that give rise to their vulnerability and lack of autonomy often result also in risk of disease and lack of access to cure.

Vaccines or drugs for diseases that affect particularly the vulnerable should be separately tested on them, to assure safety and effectiveness. Ideally this should be combined with or followed by operations research to assess the cost and feasibility of the eventual use of the product at the service of the vulnerable.[3]

Rights to informed consent

Once it is ethically responsible on the basis of equity, beneficence and non-maleficence to include or even focus on vulnerable people among the subjects of research, the question arises of how to protect them and their rights during the research.

As a base for informed consent, the same ethical principles should apply to vulnerable populations (macro-ethics) as to vulnerable subjects (micro-ethics).

The first principle underlying informed consent is respect. Many groups in the first and second categories are aware of their vulnerability and are more or less organized as communities. They are typically nomads, refugees, low castes, or occupational groups from such communities. Sometimes also women, adolescents, migrants, handicapped people and prisoners have formal or informal community structures and leaders. All expect respect for themselves as people and therefore for their community leaders; often they even feel that the researchers together with these community leaders should clear any research activity with local authorities such as those responsible for interior and health affairs.

In such cases, the first step is to identify community leaders from information provided by vulnerable persons. The second step is to arrange for discussions with these leaders to inform them about the research, to answer their questions, and to seek advice on how to select and protect subjects from their communities. Only after clear, unambiguous consent has been obtained from community leaders should local-government authorities be approached for clearance. Finally, individual informed consent can be sought, usually after more group meetings where prospective subjects are informed by community leaders and researchers and can exercise their rights to question and make suggestions. Questions and suggestions in group meetings are more likely when leaders take only a moderate advocacy role at the outset and encourage people to speak up so that no doubts or objections remain unanswered. Leaders should thus become aware of a community's feelings and suggestions and better able to represent the views of prospective subjects.

By going through these stages, investigators can be satisfied that individual consent is fully informed in a way in which it otherwise could not be. If some community members are literate they can be asked to write reports on what happened at each of the rounds of meetings. Should individual consent be similarly documented? Maybe that decision can safely be left to the community group or its leaders or both.

Vulnerable categories that are not organized as groups pose a much more difficult problem, particularly those of the first category (capable of informed consent but not accorded the right to autonomy), the second category (those unfamiliar with modern medical concepts), and the fourth category (groups dependent upon researchers). Researchers can stimulate *ad hoc* organization of those eligible for selection, which increases the chances of group discussion and a deeper exploration of the information before going on to individual consent.

Vulnerable subjects of the third category, namely those incapable of informed consent, pose the greatest challenge. They should be considered for research only when there is no genuine alternative,[4] such as when children are needed for research into conditions that affect only children. It is often considered sufficient to obtain informed consent from their legal guardians, but this practice has too often permitted abuses, as too many people and societies do not respect sufficiently the lives of these vulnerable individuals. There seems to be a general perception that these categories are not at all capable of informed consent, but in fact children become capable of it at different rates in different societies; some societies recognize them as capable of moral judgement and therefore possibly of informed consent at the age of 7 years, others at 12 or 15, and others at 18. Similarly, moderately retarded individuals or mentally ill patients or anxious-depressive individuals can give informed consent if they are permitted sufficient unpressured exploration and reflexion. Strict, globally applicable, rules regarding informed consent in this category are not possible, but it should be a special responsibility of ethical review committees to judge not only whether the proposed study meets strict ethical criteria, but also whether the procedures for obtaining informed consent maximizes the protection of these prospective subjects and their potential for autonomy.

Micro-ethics, macro-ethics and meta-ethics

The micro-ethics of research involving vulnerable subjects is embedded in the macro-ethics that refers to vulnerable groups. Whenever research focuses on vulnerable subjects only, macro-ethics becomes even a dominant concern, in particular as regards the maximizing of benefit and the minimizing of harm to the group (see International Guidelines for Ethical Review of Epidemiological Studies).

Simply to review the headings of these epidemiological guidelines (nos. 13-25) — communication of study results (to vulnerable groups); release of study results that are of public interest; training local health personnel (in relevant skills); causing harm or doing wrong to vulnerable groups, especially by harmful publicity or insensitivity to different cultures or social mores — is to realize that many researchers familiar with micro-ethics have not a clear understanding, let alone the necessary skills, of macro- or meta-ethics.

Ethical review committees beyond review

So far, ethical review by committees seems a priori, based on statements of intent. Is this enough in the case of vulnerable research subjects? It is suggested that two further mechanisms be created: an ombudsman and a watchdog. The ethical committee should be the ombudsman of groups or individuals who feel that their rights have been infringed by design or by the behaviour of researchers or their agents. This facility should be accessible even to those not categorized as vulnerable. As watchdog, an ethical committee would recognize that, beyond intent, much depends on the researcher's ethical conscience and understanding, and skill in communication. Therefore, for all research involving, in part or exclusively, vulnerable populations or subjects, it would be appropriate for ethical review committees to closely monitor informed consent procedures, the relationships of researchers to subjects, and the occurrence of harmful side-effects. Such close monitoring, carried out scientifically and systematically, should limit abuses, but also, through experiential learning, result in more refined ethical guidelines for maximizing protection and increasing autonomy.

Serious consideration should be given to the possibility that, both nationally and internationally, courses in ethics should be organized for researchers and committee members, emphasizing, beyond principles, skills in ethical problem-solving and in the recognition and protection of vulnerable groups and subjects.

This should advance greatly the practice of ethics and avoid legalistic rigidity, which is an ever present danger when ethics seems complex and those who make ethical judgements freeze in an ethical-legalistic ritual rather than perform a consequentialist life-giving ballet. It should lead to the practice of meta-ethics, in which different disciplines as well as community members would participate, becoming a reality also in the developing world.[5] It should promote normative evolutionary ethics, sensitive to people's norms and to the norms which CIOMS and others propagate as universal, and continuously watchful for consequences for study subjects and members of their groups. National or regional ethical review committees may play their part by undertaking to increase public consciousness of the rights of vulnerable groups and individuals.

References

1. Council for International Organizations of Medical Sciences, 1991, *International Guidelines for Ethical Review of Epidemiological Studies*. Geneva, CIOMS.
2. Council for International Organizations of Medical Sciences, 1991, *Ethics and Epidemiology: International Guidelines*: Proceedings of the XXVth CIOMS Conference. Geneva, CIOMS.
3. Gostin, L., 1991, Macro-Ethical Principles for the Conduct of Research on Human Subjects, in: Z. Bankowski, J.H. Bryant & J.M. Last (eds.), *Ethics and Epidemiology: International Guidelines*, Geneva, CIOMS, pp. 29-45, especially pp. 35-36.
4. Levine, R.J., 1988, *Ethics and Regulation of Clinical Research*, 2nd ed. New Haven: Yale University Press.
5. *Ethics, Humanity, Rights and AIDS in Africa*. An International Communiqué by the African AIDS Research Network (West and Central African Zone), Lagos, Nigeria, 5-7 November 1991.

DISTINGUISHING "EXPLOITABLE" FROM "VULNERABLE" POPULATIONS: WHEN CONSENT IS NOT THE ISSUE

W.K. Mariner*

Last week I heard on the radio a lengthy interview with a woman from an AIDS education organization in Philadelphia, in the United States. She befriended people who use drugs and taught them how to sterilize their needles to avoid getting HIV infection. She also taught prostitutes how to get their clients to use condoms to protect themselves from HIV infection. Many of the people she saw were African-Americans from the inner city — a population that many people in the research community would call vulnerable.

The AIDS educator said a remarkable thing. She said that many of the African-Americans she talked with were skeptical about her message about how to prevent AIDS. They told her they did not believe what the government said about condoms or bleaching needles. And why not? Because of Tuskegee. In 1932, the United States Public Health Service began a research study of more than 400 black men to learn the natural history of syphilis. They were told that they would receive special free treatment, but were not told that they were part of a research study. When penicillin was found to cure syphilis, they were not told that either, and were not given the medicine. They went to their doctor-investigators regularly but nothing was done for them until they died. The study did not become public knowledge until 1972.

The Tuskegee study is a powerful symbol of unethical research. Its memory is very much alive today. African-Americans felt betrayed, and they were right. So, even now, many African-American communities do not trust what the government tells them, even when the government is telling the truth. The memory of Tuskegee has prevented people from learning how to protect themselves against HIV infection in ways that are not at all experimental, but well established. The lesson is that unethical research can damage people in longlasting ways. If their trust has been abused by investigators, standard preventive methods, let alone research, may never again be acceptable to them.

Trends toward Expanding the Use of Vulnerable Populations

We meet at a time when there is controversy over whether the function of ethical principles is to *protect* human subjects against the risks of research, or to assure them participation in the benefits of research. Ethical guidelines themselves may be responsible for some of the confusion. There has been a shift in attitudes toward ethical research,

* Associate Professor of Health Law, School of Public Health, School of Medicine, Boston University, Boston, Massachusetts, U.S.A.

from viewing research as acceptable only with the consent of the subject to viewing research as acceptable without the subject's consent when the research proposal is reviewed by an independent body. The Nuremberg Code (Code) says that the voluntary consent of the subject is essential. The Code emphasized protecting the rights of the individual subject. In contrast, the Declaration of Helsinki and the 1982 WHO/CIOMS Proposed International Guidelines for Biomedical Research Involving Human Subjects (1982 WHO/CIOMS Guidelines) consider the welfare of the subject first priority. They would protect subjects' welfare by having an independent committee review the research before it begins, and then permit subjects to be involved without their consent if their welfare is adequately protected.

More recently, in the United States, there has been been a trend in the opposite direction — toward substituting the consent of the subject for any prior determination that the risks and benefits justify the research itself. For example, some AIDS activists have questioned the need for protecting the welfare of people with HIV infection against any risk of research, on the ground that the individual subject should be able to decide, as a matter of autonomy, what risks he or she is willing to take in the search for a cure for AIDS. Women in the United States have also argued that their traditional exclusion from research deprives them of the benefits of biomedical advances.

In this view, contrary to all existing ethical principles, the consent of the subject is sufficient to justify any research. Historically, the concept of autonomy protected the right of people to avoid the risks of research. Here, it is used to claim entitlement to the benefits of research.

Both these shifts have made it easier to use vulnerable and exploitable populations in biomedical research. Sometimes this is a good thing, as when investigators tested oral rehydration therapy and found a simple, inexpensive means to treat life-threatening diarrheal diseases in children. Sometimes, however, it is not so good. Consider, for example, the testing of the useless drug FLV-23-A on orphans with AIDS in a children's hospital in Bucharest, Romania.

I sit on an independent review committee to protect research subjects. Sometimes, investigators say that, if the committee insists on careful compliance with ethical principles, the research will be too difficult and they will "have" to do the research in Mexico or Thailand. In one instance, an investigator told the committee chairperson that he would not ask the committee to review one part of a study because the investigator knew it would not meet the committee's ethical standards; instead, the study would be conducted in South America, where the investigator believed the same standards did not have to be met. Investigators sometimes conduct research in the developing world because they think that ethical guidelines do not apply there, and often they do not apply. In part, this may be because investigators are unfamiliar with ethical principles, but it is also because the Declaration of Helsinki and the 1982 WHO/CIOMS Guidelines imply that research is so important and desirable that even vulnerable populations can be used without their consent as long as the research is reviewed by an independent body.

Remembering all the Ethical Principles of Research

Unfortunately, not all research is important and desirable. Therefore, it is always necessary to ensure that a specific research study satisfies the basic ethical principles that: (1) the research is necessary to accomplish an important goal for the benefit of society; (2) the information cannot be obtained in any other way; (3) the foreseeable benefits outweigh the possible risks to the subjects, and the risks themselves are not serious; and (4) only qualified investigators will conduct the study, conforming to a scientifically valid study design. No one — not investigators and not subjects — can waive these prerequisites.

Two other elements have been deemed necessary for ethical research: (a) that the subjects selected are both necessary and appropriate to obtaining the necessary information; and (b) that each subject voluntarily consents to participate in the research. The first, the principle of equitable subject selection, is implicit (although not always made explicit) in most ethical guidelines in the requirement that the information cannot be obtained in any other way, including from other people. All guidelines, however, deal explicitly with the subject's consent.

The Declaration of Helsinki and the 1982 WHO/CIOMS Guidelines differ from the Nuremberg Code and the Statement of the Ministers of the Council of Europe, for example, in providing that the voluntary consent of the subject *may* be waived. It is possible to justify waiving the requirement of subject consent in the case of populations who are vulnerable because of legal incapacity to consent to research or because of inability to make a choice. In those cases, proxy consent is possible.

The same is *not* true for populations that are at risk of exploitation. The 1982 WHO/CIOMS Guidelines permit investigators to obtain indirectly the "adequately informed consent of subjects" in such populations through the intermediary of a trusted community leader when the prospective subjects "do not have the necessary awareness of the implications of participation in an experiment to give adequately informed consent directly to investigators."

This provision is sometimes interpreted to mean that it is acceptable to use exploitable populations for *any* research as long as some community representative gives substitute consent, and that the only problem with using such people as subjects is getting some form of proxy consent. But surely this would be wrong. Populations are at risk of exploitation, not because they are incapable of giving consent (although some have this problem, too), but because some research would use them as means to an end, and to use them in that way would be both unjust and disrespectful of them as persons.

People tend to be considered "vulnerable" for one of two reasons: (1) they lack the capacity to give voluntary consent, or (2) they are at risk of exploitation by research. Of course, some people may be vulnerable for both reasons. Nevertheless, these reasons raise different ethical questions. The case of people who are vulnerable because they are at risk of exploitation raises the question of justice or equitable selection of subjects: whether it is just to use them as subjects of research. The case of people who are vulnerable because they cannot give voluntary consent raises both the question of justice in the selection of subjects and the further question of consent.

The Declaration of Helsinki and the 1982 WHO/CIOMS Guidelines tend to conflate these two populations. As a result, they encourage disregard for the threshold questions in research: should this research be done at all, and, if so, is it possible only in this population?

Distinguishing between Vulnerable and Exploitable Populations

We should take advantage of the opportunity to revise the 1982 WHO/CIOMS Guidelines to rethink what we mean by vulnerable populations, and how and why they should be protected. I propose distinguishing between categories of vulnerability in order to make clear that the principle of equitable selection of subjects must be satisfied *before* considering questions of consent.

I propose to limit the term "vulnerable populations" to the category of people who lack the capacity to give voluntary consent. I shall call the second category of people "exploitable populations," for lack of a better term, because they are at risk of being used as means for the ends of others.

I. Vulnerable populations

Vulnerable populations may be divided into four categories on the basis of the reason for which they are unable to give consent. The concept of consent to research is derived from the first principle of the Nuremberg Code, which requires the voluntary consent of every subject of research:

1. The voluntary consent of the human subject is absolutely essential. This means that the person involved should have legal capacity to give consent; should be so situated as to be able to exercise free power of choice, without the intervention of any element of force, fraud, deceit, duress, over-reaching, or other ulterior form of constraint or coercion; and should have sufficient knowledge and

comprehension of the elements of the subject matter involved as to enable him to make an understanding and enlightened decision.

The first principle of the Nuremberg Code is a useful statement of the four prerequisites of voluntary consent. The first is *legal capacity* or competence to give consent. The second is *voluntariness* or freedom from coercion, fraud or deceit. The third is the receipt of *information* sufficient to permit a knowledgeable choice, or the *informed* element of informed consent, which I shall refer to as the ability to make a choice. The last prerequisite is *understanding*, or comprehension of the relevant information. A person who lacks any one of these prerequisites cannot give valid consent to become a research subject.

A. Legal incapacity

People may be incompetent to consent to become a research subject either because they are denied the legal capacity to consent by law, or are mentally or physically incapable of making or communicating a decision. The classic examples of legal incapacity are children below the legal age of majority, fetuses, and people who have been declared legally incompetent by a court or other lawful entity. In addition, people who are unconscious or in a coma are incompetent to make decisions for themselves. Legal incapacity may be either temporary or permanent for the individual person.

This subcategory has the advantage that it can be defined objectively. There are obvious difficulties in deciding at what age a child should be entitled to make legal decisions concerning research, since not all children of the same age are equally capable. Nonetheless, once the decision is made, it is a relatively simple matter to apply.

B. Ability to make a choice

This subcategory rarely receives attention in discussions of vulnerable populations, because it pertains primarily to the duty of the investigator rather than to the capacity of the prospective subject. The investigator is obligated to provide sufficient information to permit a subject to make a knowledgeable decision. However, it presumes that a subject is at least capable of making a decision. Thus, it requires that people have sufficient powers of comprehension and reasoning to appreciate the information provided and make a choice.

People who are legally competent to make their own decisions may not, in fact, be able to do so. Examples include people whose powers of reasoning are impaired by medication or by the abuse of alcohol or other substances, or who are mentally or emotionally distraught. Lack of the ability to make a choice is more often temporary than permanent. The criteria for being unable to make a choice can be defined objectively. Thus, the groups in this category can be described in general terms. However, it is sometimes difficult to determine whether a particular individual is capable of making a decision.

C. *Understanding*

The requirement that prospective research-subjects understand what they are getting into is intended to ensure that people who are capable of making an autonomous decision are actually able to make the decision they would want to make. People's capacity of understanding can be impaired by the same things that impair their powers of reasoning and designate them as vulnerable for the second reason just described. In addition, however, people who may be capable of making an informed decision may not understand what they are being asked to decide. For example, investigators may present the information in terms that the subjects do not comprehend, even though most other people would understand the same presentation. Some people do not have sufficient background or experience to appreciate what is being described.

It is difficult to identify specific groups of people as vulnerable on the ground that they lack understanding, since comprehension is specific to the individual and to the information that is presented. However, lack of understanding can sometimes be remedied by more comprehensive, simpler, and creative ways of presenting the information. Therefore, if it is justifiable to use as research subjects groups of people who might not understand technical explanations, it is essential to develop ways of presenting information so that it is comprehensible to them.

D. *Voluntariness*

This subcategory covers people whose autonomy or freedom of choice and action is compromised in some way, not by any incapacity but by circumstances external to them. Unlike the first three subcategories, individuals may be quite competent and able to understand the nature of the research and come to a knowledgeable decision. However, they may not be able to act on their decision because they are somehow forced, coerced, pressured, or tricked into doing something they would prefer not to do (or not doing something they want to do). People who are dependent on researchers or their collaborators may be improperly influenced by those in positions of authority.

The classic example of this type of population is prisoners. It also includes both adults and children who are institutionalized for other reasons. If they are institutionalized because of some mental impairment, they are vulnerable for two reasons. Not only may they not be able to understand what they are asked to do, but the institution may put overt or subtle pressure on them to participate in research. Hospital patients fall into this category, because they may feel too dependent for care upon their physicians or the institution to refuse any offer.

One need not be institutionalized to be vulnerable for reasons of involuntariness, however. Employees may be induced to participate in research by promises of favorable treatment or less congenially by threats of losing their jobs if they do not enroll. Employees of researchers, including research assistants and medical, nursing, and dental students, may feel unable to say "no" to their superiors.

The characteristics of circumstances that compromise autonomy and threaten involuntariness can be defined objectively, although actual situations may vary slightly from culture to culture. However, some individuals in even involuntary circumstances are fully capable of withstanding intimidation and making voluntary decisions.

E. Summary of discussion on vulnerable populations

When one of these populations is proposed as subjects for research, the first question is whether it is justifiable to use them as subjects at all. Under the Nuremberg Code, no vulnerable population could be used, because the consent of each subject is absolutely necessary. The Code recognized, however, that some vulnerable populations are subject to unique diseases or conditions that should be cured or ameliorated; common examples are diseases unique to childhood and mental illnesses. It would be difficult to know whether new medicines or biomedical techniques could help such diseases without testing them on such groups. Also, some groups may have special genetic characteristics that affect the safety and effectiveness of medicines and biomedical techniques; in such circumstances, a justifiable exception can be made to the prohibition against using vulnerable populations as subjects of research. This justification has three important limitations: First, the purpose of the research must be to benefit the vulnerable population used as research subjects. Second, it must be scientifically impossible to obtain the desired information without the participation of the vulnerable population. Third, the research must be so clearly in the best interests of the individual research-subjects that they would voluntarily agree to participate if they were capable of giving valid consent.

Where these requirements are satisfied, the research itself is important and justifiable and the principle of equitable selection of subjects is observed. It may be presumed that the vulnerable population would want to participate. The only problem is how to carry out what may be considered the reasonable wishes of the population. Thus, we reach the second ethical question — that of consent. The problem is resolved by using proxy consent — that is, by having another person speak for the prospective subject.

It is important to note that proxy consent applies only in the case of the first two subcategories of vulnerable populations: those who lack the legal capacity to consent, and those who lack the ability to make a choice. This is because they are incapable of making a decision, so someone else must speak for them.

However, proxy consent is difficult to justify for the third and fourth subcategories — those who lack understanding and those whose freedom is compromised. This is because they are fully capable of making a decision. Something else hinders them from making the decision they would want to make. In the case of populations that may not understand the information presented, the remedy is to improve the way in which information is presented. Those whose freedom is compromised so that they cannot made decisions voluntarily present a different question: are they better served by permitting the participation of those who can in fact make a voluntary decision, or by precluding the participation of the entire population in order to avoid mistakenly including someone who is not in fact acting voluntarily.

II. Exploitable populations

What I have called "exploitable populations" does not raise the question of consent. Exploitable populations are at risk of being used as a means to someone else's ends, of being exploited by the conduct of research. Exploitable populations differ from vulnerable populations in that they are quite capable of giving competent, voluntary, informed and understanding consent. Some exploitable populations may not have the capacity for voluntary consent, but this means that they may be classified as vulnerable in addition to exploitable. Exploitable populations cause concern *not* because of any inherent incapacity in the people themselves, but because investigators could misuse them.

Rural, non-industrialized, and illiterate communities in the developing world are perhaps the most commonly cited examples of what I call exploitable populations. In the developed world, poor urban or rural communities with limited access to the fruits of development would also qualify as exploitable populations. Dr De Sweemer-Ba in her paper points out that groups can be marginalized, and therefore subject to exploitation by virtue of social injustice, such as lack of access to food and water, or discrimination on the basis of race, class, caste, ancestry, disease, physical condition, or occupation. Other exploitable populations include people who are seriously or terminally ill and pregnant women. Some researchers may prey upon the hopes and fears of people with fatal illnesses to induce them to test useless drugs or devices for their disease. Pregnant women could be used as a vehicle to test drugs or procedures that are intended to benefit solely the fetus and offer no benefit to the women themselves. In some cultures, women who are legally or customarily subservient to their fathers or husbands may be manipulated to serve the ends of others. Some institutionalized groups, such as prisoners and mental-hospital patients, have been used because they are a convenient and inexpensive "captive audience."

In all these circumstances, the motivation of the researcher may be called into question. Regardless of the faith that investigators may have in their research, if they select an exploitable population simply for convenience to get the research done, the population is at risk of exploitation. People are being used as means, not ends, in violation of the ethical principle of respect for persons.

The risk of exploitation is also an issue of social justice. The question presented by exploitable populations is not *whether* they can give consent, and it is not *how* consent can be obtained. It is not a matter of consent at all. It is whether they should be used as research subjects at all. This question cannot be answered by saying, for example, that the community or a community leader can consent for them.

Thus, it is important to determine first whether a population is exploitable and therefore whether it is justifiable to use such a population as research subjects. If it is justifiable, the question of whether the population is incapable of consenting and therefore vulnerable is reached. The way in which such questions might be asked and answered is illustrated in Figure 1.

There are circumstances in which members of exploitable populations could justifiably be used as research subjects. These are the same circumstances as those that justify using vulnerable populations in research: that the research is intended to develop a way to ameliorate a condition unique to that population, and it cannot be accomplished by using any other population (because of genetic, physiological, or environmental differences that affect the results). One might also add that it would be difficult to justify conducting research on an exploitable population unless the benefits of successful research became available to the population.

A contemporary example from the United States is communities of gay men. HIV-positive gay men could be considered an exploitable population because they are at risk of exploitation from promoters of useless nostrums and regimens touted as life-prolonging. However, the AIDS epidemic calls for unusual speed in finding ways to relieve or cure AIDS and HIV-related illnesses. Some experimental products with scientific promise can be tested only with people who are HIV-positive; and, if effective, the research would benefit the subject population. Finally, the majority of the gay community in the United States are educated, middle-class males who are familiar with health care and medical research. Therefore, the ethical principle of just subject-selection is satisfied. It is justifiable to test certain drugs, for example, in an otherwise exploitable population. Moreover, there is no problem with consent. This population is not vulnerable. Most members are fully capable of making a competent, voluntary,

Figure 1

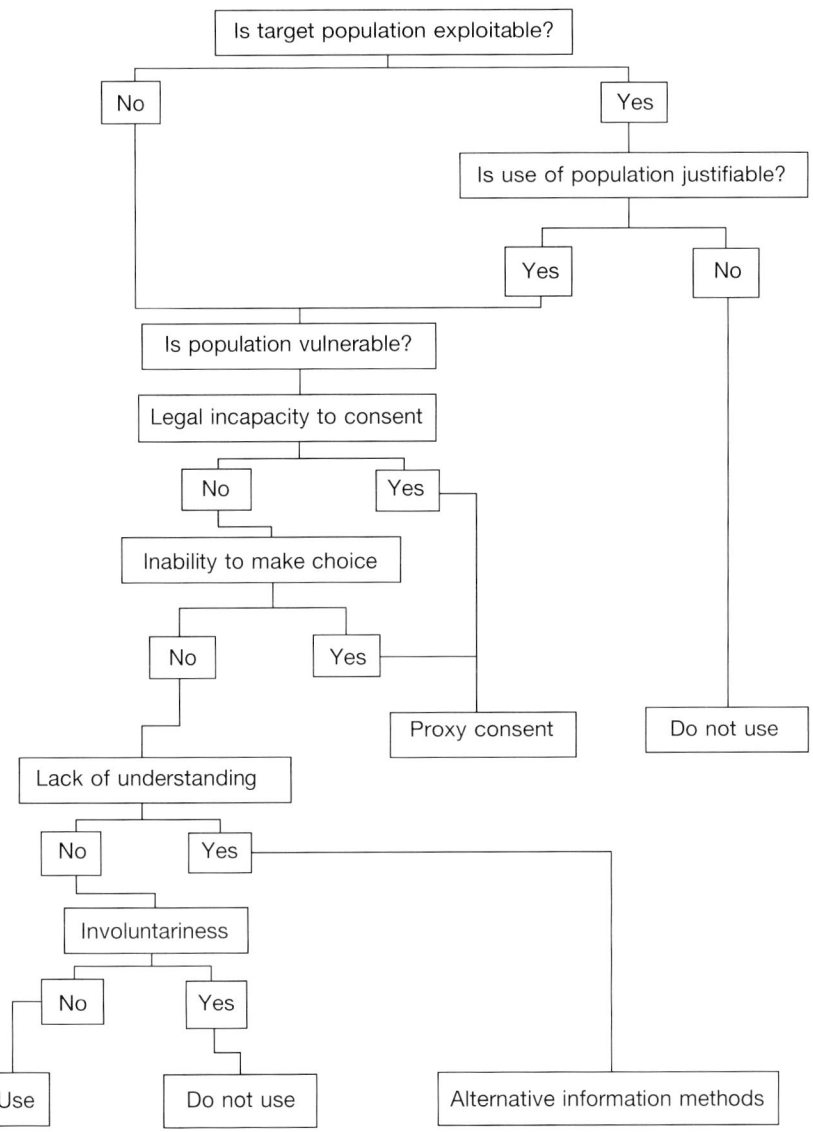

informed, and understanding decision about becoming a research subject.

Other reasons to include exploitable populations in research

Are there other reasons to include exploitable populations in research? Recently, it has been claimed that such populations should be used as research subjects because *not* using them would deprive them of some benefit. The validity of this argument depends upon whether research is considered to be a benefit in and of itself. The judges who expounded the Nuremberg Code viewed research as suspect, potentially dangerous. The 1982 WHO/CIOMS Guidelines, in contrast, view research as good.

The 1982 Guidelines state that "the Nuremberg Code ... [has] been superseded by 'Helsinki'." This is, of course, incorrect. The Declaration of Helsinki was drafted by physicians and researchers for their own use in *biomedical* research. It does not concern other kinds of research. Critics of Helsinki argue that it was intended to get around the Nuremberg Code's insistence on the voluntary consent of each subject. Supporters argue that it was designed to address issues of therapeutic medical research that were definitely not at issue in the Nazi doctors' trial at Nuremberg. There is truth in both arguments. But the judgment that included the Nuremberg Code still stands and the Code's principles remain valid. The 1990 Recommendation of the Committee of Ministers of the Council of Europe sounds more like the Nuremberg Code than the Helsinki Declaration, and it covers more than biomedical research.

Like the Declaration of Helsinki, the 1982 Guidelines deal only with biomedical research. Biomedical research is supposed to provide generalized knowledge that will improve human health and welfare. Therefore, when we speak of the Guidelines, it is easy to assume that we are dealing only with research that will benefit humankind. It is also easy to believe that such research will produce only benefits. Indeed, I doubt that any investigator could conduct research without believing that it would produce a benefit. Thus, it is also easy to believe that people would want to be part of research in order to obtain those benefits.

Those who believe that research is good may also believe that the burden is on others to prove that the research will harm the subjects more than it benefits them or others. For those who consider research to be potentially dangerous, the burden is on the researchers and sponsors to prove that specific populations should be used as research subjects. Which approach should we adopt? Although I believe that most biomedical research is good, I know that not all of it is good. More important, the benefits that people desire from research do not always reach them. Therefore, it is wiser to require researchers to bear the burden of proving that it is necessary to use a specific population as research subjects. With this approach, virtually all good research is justifiable. With the opposite approach, there is a significant danger that harmful research will be permitted along with the good.

Conclusion

I began this presentation with a story that ended with a warning: if we allow unethical research to harm an exploitable population, we may cause irreparable damage both to the population of research subjects and to the enterprise of research itself. As we look forward to a new generation of ethical principles, let us remember the reasons for having ethical principles in the first place: to protect people from harm. Distinguishing exploitable from vulnerable populations may help us to do that by reminding us to ask the right question: Is there a valid scientific reason why these are the only people that can serve as research subjects? If the answer is yes, then and only then may we consider whether they are capable of consent, and, if not, whether proxy consent is justified.

REPORT OF WORKING GROUP A: INFORMED CONSENT

Moderator: **J.M. Last**
Rapporteur: **R.J. Cook** and **K.S. Khan**

Group A discussed the topic of informed consent under a series of questions formulated by the conference organizers, and the report is constructed on the basis of the questions.

1. *In communities where there is not a tradition of individual consent, can reliance be placed on agreement of community leaders?*

The group's consensus was that agreement of community leaders may not be used in place of informed consent, or as a short-cut, to pursue biomedical research. Obtaining informed consent protects the research subject's freedom of choice and respects individual autonomy. In addition, in communities where research is new or has not been undertaken, it is important to develop a community forum where the purposes of the research can be explained and debated.

Respect for persons is an inviolable condition of all research involving human subjects. Regardless of the position of the person in the collective to which the person belongs, whether that collective is a nuclear family, a clan, tribe, community or nation, if the person is the unit of study that person must be respected. This applies even though there may be a designated "head", "leader", "spokesman" for the collective, and even though this designated "head" may authorize the research. Nevertheless, the opinions or beliefs of the collective should be respected also.

In communities where women do not have the authority to be self-determining, such as where they have no or limited legal capacity, or where it is customary to secure husbands' authorization for research instead of the informed consent of women, every effort should be made to secure the informed consent of women no matter how difficult it might be to do so. Suggestions as to how best to explain the information to bring about the understanding necessary for informed consent included dialogue with groups who were traditionally disfranchised, to permit abstract concepts related to research to be explained in ways that such groups could understand. In dealing with disfranchised women the objective of the process of informed consent is to enable them to become more self-determining.

2. *How and by whom may an investigator be authorized to conduct biomedical research in communities where there is little or no tradition of research or prospective ethical review of research?*

There was strong consensus that only ethical review committees should be authorized to approve biomedical research. It was recognized, however, that for many communities this remained the ideal, and specific suggestions were made as to how to make the ideal a reality. They included the establishment of training programmes in bioethics, and ensuring that scientific and medical journals did not accept articles based on research done without prior ethical review and without the informed and voluntary consent of the research subjects.

It was pointed out that under Article 7 of the International Covenant on Civil and Political Rights "... no one shall be subjected without his free consent to medical or scientific experimentation."

3. *How may the legitimacy of material and other inducements to participate in research be assessed?*

Regarding inducements, rewards, incentives to become a research subject (and to do research), standards and values differ sharply according to sociocultural and economic conditions. No firm or fixed rules seem possible.

There was no disagreement about reimbursing patients for expenses, including time spent away from work, of being a research subject. Concern was expressed about other inducements to undergo research, such as fraudulent information about the benefits of research, particularly among such vulnerable groups as leprosy patients, pregnant women and prostitutes. Consent obtained through fraudulent information about benefits would be totally invalid.

The group distinguished between inducements to research subjects to join research and inducements to investigators. It was agreed that offers, financial or other, that overcame a person's ability to give free consent were illegitimate; that offers of compensation to research subjects should cover actual costs and work-time lost; and that such compensation should be mentioned in the research proposal submitted for approval to the ethical review committee. Any reward in cash or kind to the researcher, or to the researcher's department or institution, must be declared and considered as subject to the ethical review.

4. *What should be the limits on the authority of legal guardians or responsible relatives to grant permission for the participation of vulnerable individuals?*

Limits on guardians' authority often exist in law, but the law almost invariably lets guardians approve procedures that are therapeutically intended, and may indeed require guardians to approve such procedures. However, the law may limit guardians' powers to approve non-therapeutically intended procedures on those under their care. The law may limit guardians' powers to approve invasive procedures on vulnerable persons, but permit such non-invasive procedures as weighing, measuring, and urine testing for non-therapeutically intended purposes (i.e., purposes that have no therapeutic value to the research subjects).

Some vulnerable persons, such as "street kids", who live in communities of their own kind or in isolation have no adult guardians. They may be invited to participate in research that offers them some immediate health benefit, but care must be taken not to induce them to take part in other studies by offering the prospect of adult companionship or protection. Means must be found to inform their communities of what is proposed and to explain proposals to the peer group.

5. *What limits should there be to the autonomy of the following groups to consider participation in research? (i) Women who are a) pregnant; b) lactating; c) biologically capable of conception; (ii) Men who are biologically capable of initiating conception.*

The initial presumption that all competent persons can make their own decisions lays the burden of proof on anyone who proposes limits on the research to which a competent person can consent. Fertility is not a basis of loss of choice to be a research subject. Exclusion criteria of autonomous choice to enter studies should rest on proven scientific evidence from human or relevant animal studies of harm to children in excess of the ordinary risk of harm among children in the population it is proposed to study.

6. *Are there any other vulnerable groups that should be given special protection?*

Groups at special risk are recognized. These are variously described as "vulnerable", "exploited" (or "exploitable"), "disfranchised", "minorities", "underclass". Members of these groups may be at higher risk than others of being harmed by research. Ethical review must pay particular attention to the special needs of persons who belong to such groups. They may be in special need of help from an ombudsman, patient advocate or other "watchdog". Examples of such groups include homeless people, periurban slum dwellers, nomads, refugees, recent immigrants, and persons with diseases that carry a social stigma.

Some individuals are vulnerable, not because of inability to understand information relevant to consent, but because they do not feel free to deny consent; examples are students and employees. They warrant being protected against their exploitability. Others are vulnerable because they lack ability to understand information that research subjects are entitled to receive. Criteria should be established to identify individuals' liability to exploitation, such as through dependence on investigators, poverty, refugee status or isolation from a family or community or other lack of support of others, and subjects of unjust social structures. Exploitable individuals may not be members of predictable categories, and investigators need to take great care in regard to proposals to undertake studies among collectivities of persons who seem liable to exploitation because of their dependency and need to defer to others' preferences.

7. *Should the Guidelines provide for sanctions against studies performed without consent or with fraudulently obtained consent?*
The Guidelines should indicate sanctions that could be applied, and who should bear responsibility for ensuring investigators' answerability for ethical misconduct (e.g., ethical review committee, employer, sponsor or funding agency, professional association, disciplinary committee). Options include delicensure, legal sanctions such as criminal penalties for assault or fraud, and sanctions by human rights tribunals at domestic or international levels. For instance, when state-organized institutions have collaborated in a tolerated impropriety, action may be initiated if the state is a party to the International Covenant on Civil and Political Rights. (See also Report of Working Group B, item 9.)

* * *

The discussion on informed consent highlighted some fundamental issues on which it was thought the Guidelines might need to take unequivocal positions. These are:

1. Whereas the Guidelines seek to balance the rights of potential research subjects (as individual human beings) with the rights of researchers, they should leave no doubt as to whether ultimately it is the right of the research subject that is to be protected or that of the researcher. If the concern for the research subject is central, then it becomes the reference point for all other principles, even if it means encroaching upon the researcher's right. Thus the question is: whose rights are the more important?

2. On the issue of competency/incompetency to give consent, a strong case was made for nearly anybody with the competency to give consent to do so, provided time, patience and different approaches were adopted (Exceptions in such cases would be few).

   It was suggested that the Conference needed to take a position on whether competency to give consent was to be adopted as a primary principle, with incompetency to be relegated only to, for example, infants, or to be entirely ruled out, even in the form of proxy consent.

3. The meanings of certain key terms needed to be stated precisely — for example, research; therapeutic and non-therapeutic research; experiment; biomedical; vulnerable; exploited; underclass; informed or uninformed consent; and purpose of research, i.e., relevant to whom and why (especially in relation to countries where health services are disorganized). Also, the wording of different principles and guidelines should be examined minutely to point out ambiguities or invite clarification.

4. Is the concept of research-subjects' rights in consonance with the concept of right as enunciated by the International Covenant on Civil and Political Liberties (Article 7)?

5. A clear differentiation should be made between the research subject as a patient and the research subject as a non-patient.

6. The Guidelines cannot assume the existence as well as the integrity of ethical review committees in all countries.

7. Are the Guidelines like laws to be strictly followed, or are they intended to help determine whether research practices violate the fundamental human rights of research subjects?

8. How could the Guidelines be ultimately written, e.g., in language that is easily understandable by lay people, such as that of the Universal Declaration of Human Rights?

9. On the issue of prisoners as research subjects, their fundamental right as human beings, despite the restriction on their free movement in society, needs to be first clearly stated as acceptable or not, before deliberating about their right to be research subjects.

10. Finally, it seems that there is a need to state that the Guidelines can neither assume that all researchers are suspected of violating human rights nor ignore the grave possibility of abuse of human beings. The Guidelines are designed to protect the rights of research subjects by invoking the responsibility of researchers to respect the rights of research subjects, and alerting the research subjects and the public to the rights of research subjects.

Group A raised broader issues that were not being specifically addressed by any specific guidelines:

1. Would it be useful to have a typology of research so that the issue of informed consent could be addressed in greater or less detail on the basis of the type of research to be conducted, who are likely to be the research subjects, and where the research will be conducted? This could help deal with the situation where either there are no ethical review procedures or they are ineffective.

   The basis of categorization of research was not sufficiently discussed.

2. Should the Guidelines take the position that without individual consent no research will be conducted?

3. What is the ultimate purpose of the Guidelines? In other words, it may be unequivocally said that they are meant to protect the individual research-subject from the 'group' to which he or the

belongs if there is a possibility of that 'group' considering the individual's autonomy to be secondary (Women, for example, could be the individuals within the family or community); and also to protect the group (as possible research subjects) from an individual who could use the group as a means to his or her end (the individual here being the researcher or the community leader). However, it may need to be said clearly that ultimately the Guidelines must protect the research subject.

4. Should it be said that research is good in itself and therefore the Guidelines strive to delineate the conditions that would facilitate research? Or should the Guidelines take the position that research is good in so far as it does not take advantage of an exploitable group and that it is a means of promoting human well-being but without using exploitable groups as means to that end?

5. How can the Guidelines address (or accommodate) the vulnerability of research subjects when their vulnerability is predicated on the very dynamics of their society, i.e., a society without ethical review procedures and without a properly funtioning judicial system or with dilapidated health services? In other words, can the Guidelines provide space to concerned individuals/groups in an unjust society to work for safeguarding the rights of research subjects?

6. What would constitute unethical research? If health services are grossly inadequate, and there is no mechanism for improving them or there is lack of political will to improve people's health, and therefore any research findings are not likely to contribute to health services (or systems) development, would research in such conditions be considered unethical?

ETHICAL REVIEW PROCEDURES

APPLICATION OF ETHICAL GUIDELINES IN NON-WESTERN CULTURES

M. Abdussalam*

Introduction

The basic elements of "respect for persons", "beneficence (or non-malificence)" and "justice", on which ethical guidelines for biomedical research are based, are universally valid. However, their application in different cultures requires adaptation of procedures to local social norms and economic conditions. Levine (1991)[1] has, for example, pointed out that the concept of "person" differs in Western and non-Western cultures so much that it influences the nature of "informed consent" obtained from subjects of research. Western (mainly North American) cultures emphasize individual autonomy of persons, whereas in many traditional cultures the family and even the community may have to be consulted before an individual consents to be a research subject. Levine proposes certain procedural approaches for resolving problems of informed consent in applying ethical guidelines in different cultures. The application of ethical guidelines in poor developing countries, however, requires consideration of additional factors not only to adapt to various cultures but also to overcome the negative effects of poverty, squalor and lack of education or literacy.

It should be remembered that the CIOMS Guidelines, though meant for universal application, will be used mostly by the developing countries. The industrialized countries have their own institutions and commissions for biomedical ethics and use the CIOMS Guidelines largely for research that they sponsor in developing countries.

The volume of health research is steadily increasing in many developing countries but mechanisms for ethical review are still quite weak or non-existent. Although, in the words of Osuntokun (1991),[2] "it would be naïve to expect guidelines to be quickly and effectively established in Third World countries", every effort should be made to enable these countries to apply the core elements of the Guidelines. This can be done by devising procedures suited to local sociocultural conditions, and through WHO and bilateral cooperation in building up local capacity of ethical review.

In a recent paper Professor Osuntokun and this author[3] discussed some problems of ethical review of epidemiological research in developing countries and proposed some practical approaches to overcome them. Most of these problems arise also in biomedical research involving human subjects. In the following pages some of the more important considerations applicable in conditions of under-

* Bundesgesundheitsamt, Berlin, Germany.

development are discussed on the basis of discussions which the author held recently with research and health-system managers mainly in the Eastern Mediterranean and South-East Asian countries.

Mechanisms for ethical review

Few developing countries have created independent committees for ethical review of research projects. Presumably, this function is performed by the committees that evaluate projects for scientific quality and for allocation of funds. This arrangement may be regarded as satisfactory if ethicists, jurists and lay representatives of the community are included in the membership of the committee. Lack of formal education should not bar the participation of community representatives in the committee. Such committees are generally set up by the national (central) health authority or the medical research council or an equivalent body. The committee advises not only on research projects but also on research and ethical policy, including policy on international collaborative research.

If the country is large and divided into provinces, local review committees may be set up in the provinces, universities and large research institutions. These committees can also monitor projects for the observance of ethical requirements in research work in progress.

Research-promoting agencies (bilateral and multilateral) should not forget the building up of national capacity for ethical review in their cooperation to promote essential (developmental) research and its management.

Issues of concern in the ethical review

Essential items to be reviewed in examining research projects are listed and discussed in *International guidelines for ethical review of epidemiological studies*[4] and in the present draft Guidelines. Following are brief comments on some of them from the point of view of developing countries.

(a) It is not uncommon for academics in developing countries to embark upon research that has little or only slight relevance to their countries' health problems. They may be seeking academic advancement through publication of their work in international scientific journals, which is often a condition for promotion, especially in universities. It would be unethical to subject human beings to such irrelevant research.

(b) Sometimes the preparatory laboratory and animal studies on substances and procedures to be tested in humans are omitted or only partially undertaken, on the excuse that funds and facilities are not available or inadequate. Indeed, animal experiments may be more expensive than those using human subjects. Reviewers of research protocols and supervisors should insist firmly on sufficient evidence of safety of a procedure or test before agreeing to its use on human beings.

(c) Informed consent willingly given by mentally competent subjects of research is a prerequisite stressed by various national and international codes (Nuremberg to Helsinki IV) and the CIOMS Guidelines. Reviewers should satisfy themselves that consent was obtained after explaining to the prospective subjects the nature, objectives and expected benefits of the study. Possible hazards to the subjects should be explained to them, including effects of publication of results and possible leakage of confidential information. They should be given enough time to reflect, and, if necessary, to consult their families and elders of the community.

Lack of formal education (even illiteracy) or different beliefs about disease are no bar to obtaining informed consent. With patient and judicious explanation it should be possible to fulfil all conditions of valid informed consent. If money or other material rewards are offered, they should not be in excess of normal compensation for inconvenience or time devoted. Reviewers of the research project have to be vigilant and should scrutinize the possibility of obtaining consent by excessive payment, which carries the risk of "acceptance" of serious hazards.

Subjects should be assured that they are at liberty to withdraw at any stage during the study without fear or prejudice or loss of prestige.

Some investigators obtain signed (or thumb-impressed) written statements of consent for legal purposes. From the ethical point of view these written agreements have no additional advantage or value.

The principles of obtaining consent in respect of special groups such as children, mentally retarded individuals, prisoners and condemned criminals in developing countries are the same as in other parts of the world. In some situations, however, very poor and destitute individuals or socially underprivileged groups (e.g. pariahs, untouchables, migrants) may have to be considered as vulnerable groups with restricted freedom to make truly independent choices.

(d) Provision for compensation for accidental injury to research subjects should be included in the project and reviewers should see that it is not forgotten. Apart from compensation for physical or social harm from research procedures, subjects deserve to be given health care for a disease detected during the study, even though it is not attributable to the research intervention.

Confidentiality

The confidentiality of personal data should be strictly respected. If poor people are imperfectly clad or their habitations are not completely closed to view from outside, it does not mean that they have no need for protection of personal information.

In publishing and disseminating the results of research, the anonymity of the subjects should ordinarily be protected. If this is not possible, the subject should be informed before consent to participate in the study is obtained. The consequences of self-disclosure of confidential information by the subject should also be explained before consent is obtained.

The obligation to assure confidentiality applies also to information about personal behaviour. Moreover, underhand methods, such as the use of secret observers and hidden cameras, should not be used for the collection of behavioural data.

Externally sponsored research

Many international, national and private agencies sponsor, administer or carry out health research in developing countries. Some of this work consists of testing drugs, vaccines and devices developed in industrialized countries. The volume of externally sponsored research has been increasing in many developing countries in recent years, and, if well planned and regulated, it can be mutually beneficial in promoting health research. The ethics of this type of cooperation, especially with regard to drug and vaccine testing, has been much discussed in the last decade around such key words as "ethical imperialism" and "ethical relativism".

Reviewers and other authorities should take care to ensure that such cooperative research:

— has relevance to the needs of the host country;

— does not disrupt the priorities in essential health research of the country and does not divert trained personnel from other more important tasks;

— includes training of local personnel in research methodology;

— fulfils the relevant ethical requirements of the host country as well as of the country of the sponsoring agency. (WHO has its own mechanism for ethical review of research involving human subjects.)

Conclusion

The basic ethical principles that guide biomedical research are the same throughout the world but their application in developing countries requires adaptation to local cultures and socioeconomic conditions. This can be achieved through devising suitable procedures and not by copying models of affluent industrialized countries. It is therefore important that health authorities prescribe suitable procedures and assure their application by setting up review mechanisms at central, and if necessary, peripheral levels.

References

1. Levine, R.J., 1991, Informed consent: some challenges to the universal validity of the Western model. In: Z. Bankowski, J.H. Bryant & J.M. Last (eds), *Ethics and Epidemiology: International Guidelines, CIOMS*, Geneva, pp. 47-58.
2. Osuntokun, B.O., 1991, Epidemiology and ethics, perspectives of developing countries. In: Z. Bankowski, J.H. Bryant & J.M. Last (eds), *Ethics and Epidemiology: International Guidelines*, CIOMS, Geneva, pp. 150-152.
3. Abdussalam, M. and Osuntokun, B.O., 1991, Capacity building for ethical consideration of epidemiological studies: perspective of developing countries. *Ibid.*, pp. 126-136.
4. Council for International Organizations of Medical Sciences, 1991, *International Guidelines for Ethical Review of Epidemiological Studies*. Geneva, CIOMS.

ETHICAL REVIEW PROCEDURES:
A DEVELOPED COUNTRIES' PERSPECTIVE

R. Gillon*

A Common Framework

In assessing the ethical adequacy of biomedical activities it is increasingly widely recognized that four prima facie** moral principles or values, plus attention to their scope of application, are of widespread relevance and acceptability.[1-4] These are **respect for autonomy** — an obligation to respect people's self rule or deliberated choices for themselves (autonomy literally means self-rule), insofar as such respect is compatible with an equal respect for the autonomy of all affected; **beneficence** — an obligation to help or benefit; **non-maleficence** — an obligation not to harm; and **justice or fairness** — more difficult to put in a nutshell but an obligation involving fair adjudication between competing claims, and requiring equality of treatment of those having equal claims or equal deserts (equity as distinct from mere equality of treatment), and sometimes subdivided into **justice in the context of scarce resources, justice in the context of respect for rights, and justice in the context of respect for (morally acceptable) laws**. In the case of each of these four principles there is the additional question of its scope of application: to whom or to what do we have these obligations? These principles plus attention to their scope of application do *not* provide a method for prioritising or balancing them against each other when they conflict, and so they do not provide a mechanism for making moral decisions. They do however provide a potentially international and intercultural basis for (a) a (minimal) moral commitment to certain moral values; (b) a (minimal) agreed moral language; and (c) a (minimal) framework for moral analysis.

I shall use this analytic framework in reviewing my allocated subject for this conference, namely ethical review procedures and processes, both local and national; practical impediments to adequate functioning of ethical review processes; ethical review of research with foreign sponsors; and 'capacity building' for ethical review in developing countries, as seen from the perspective of developed countries (though

---

* Imperial College of Science, Technology and Medicine and St Mary's Hospital Medical School, London, England.

** **prima facie** — a technical term introduced by the philosopher, W.D. Ross, in *The Right and the Good* (Oxford University Press, 1930, Chapter 2). Prima facie moral obligations are those that on reflection we know ourselves to have and by which we should, if there are no conflicting moral obligations, be morally bound. If there are conflicting moral obligations we need to decide which is the most important moral obligation in the particular context. The four prima facie principles do not give us a method for deciding between them or for settling such conflicts.

in this area perhaps most if not all of us are inhabitants of developing countries).

Therapeutic and Non-Therapeutic Research

Medical research may use the techniques of medicine and science to produce or try to produce benefits either for the human beings who are the subjects of that research (therapeutic research) or for the benefit of others, typically future patients (non-therapeutic research). And of course much medical research combines both intentions, in varying proportions. Both sorts of benefit are highly desirable, but patients and indeed most people are likely to assume that anything that doctors propose should be done to them will be intended for their benefit. This is the Hippocratic or therapeutic assumption that underlies all ordinary clinical practice and upon which the relationship of trust between patient and doctor is based. Where research is intended for the benefit of others, whether as well as for, or particularly instead of, the benefit of the subject, the Hippocratic assumption is nullified or modified and subjects must be made aware of that modification or nullification, and their consent to involvement must be based on such awareness. Otherwise their autonomy will be infringed, for their decision-making about whether or not to accept the doctor's proposals must, if it is to be autonomous, be based on adequate knowledge of the facts, and the doctor's attitude and intentions are for the subject vital facts in deciding what further information he or she requires; for example, how much simply to trust the doctor to make decisions on the patient's behalf ('oh well if it's what the doctor wants it must be what he or she thinks will be best for me'), or how much to be on guard against potential dangers, risks, distress and inconvenience.

It is because of this potential — perhaps inevitable — ambiguity of intention of the medical researcher (benefit for the patient/subject — the Hippocratic commitment — vs. benefit for others) that research ethics review procedures are necessary and have been developed, and this would have been true, I believe, even if there had been no human-experiment atrocities by Nazi doctors to stimulate the original Nuremberg Code on medical experimentation[5] and then the Declaration of Helsinki.[6]

Moral objectives of research ethics committees

On the basis of the above analytic framework, the moral objectives of a research ethics committee (REC) are to promote potentially beneficial medical research of a sort that protects the research subject from unjustified risk of harm; ensures respect for his or her autonomy; is scientifically valid and thus can in principle produce benefits, and is explicit about who are the intended recipients of such benefits; and meets the moral requirements of justice in terms of respect for research subjects' rights and respect for morally acceptable laws. What research ethics committees have so far explicitly rejected is any role in assessing resource implications of research proposals (the moral requirement of distributive justice). There is no reason for this to be part of the remit of a research ethics committee, but such assessment is a necessary part of a complete ethical review of research proposals and it should be made explicit (a) whose task the evaluation of the resource implications of research proposals should be, and (b) that REC approval has *not* taken into account any assessment of resource implications.

Necessary membership of research ethics committees

The membership of a research ethics committee should be designed so as to promote the above moral objectives. There is no agreed 'blueprint' for an ideal REC, but multidisciplinarity is needed to provide the range of perspectives needed. Expert medical researchers are needed to provide the expertise necessary for evaluation of the scientific validity of research proposals (though such expertise may need to be supplemented for particular proposals by the obtaining of specialized additional advice); doctors who are primarily or entirely 'therapeutic' clinicians (i.e. non-researchers) are needed to provide the Hippocratic perspective, in which the interests of the patient/subject are paramount; some nations including Britain require a non-hospital doctor (general practitioner) and also a clinical nurse to be included on RECs, to strengthen this 'subject-protecting' perspective. Above all, a *public* perspective is needed, which should include at least one respected member of the public who has no professional or institutional ties with the organization setting up the REC. In this regard the existing CIOMS guidelines are, I believe, too weak in stating (S23) that RECs are essentially peer review committees that 'may' include non-medical health professionals and laymen. In Britain both the Government's regulations for research ethics committees[7] and the much older Royal College of Physicians guidelines[8] require 'lay' representation and the same is true of American regulations.[9]

Nor does there seem to be an agreed blueprint for the number of members of a REC — again it should be sufficient to achieve its moral objectives. US regulations specify at least five members, not all men or all women, not all from a single profession, and of sufficiently diverse backgrounds 'to promote respect for its advice and counsel in safeguarding the rights and welfare of human subjects[9]. On the other hand, Dr Levine's pioneering institutional review board or IRB (the American name for a research ethics committee) had 26 members, including four medical students and one public health student.[9] In Britain the government guidelines recommend 8-12 members, from both sexes, from a wide range of age groups, with at least two 'lay persons', one totally unconnected professionally with health care and the National Health Service (NHS). Finally the British government guidelines require that the Chair and vice-Chair be appointed by the District Health Authority, which sets up the REC and appoints all its members, and that either the Chair or the vice-Chair be one of the lay members of the committee. The Royal College of Physicians guidelines recommend that the Chair and vice-Chair be elected by the committees themselves and make no such requirement that at least one must be a lay member. The CIOMS revision group may care to consider whether or not the current CIOMS guidelines should be revised so as to advise on these issues. The ethical issue seems to be primarily whether or not such requirements are necessary for the adequate protection of research subjects.

For my own part I would add a recommendation that at least one member of any REC should have 'analytic skills', of the sort that are part of the academic training of lawyers, philosophers and moral theologians. The skills I have in mind include the ability (and tendency) to scrutinize arguments, even those defending received wisdom, for flaws, and also to look for, and appreciate the strengths of, counterarguments. On the whole, the development of such skills has not typically comprised part of the training of health care professionals but it does seem needed for rigorous moral analysis.

Should committees sit in public or in private?

American regulations (for federally funded research) do not require rights of public access, but Dr Levine reports that the Yale University IRB meetings are open to the public (though not advertised as such)[9] (p. 217,). English RECs meet in private and their proceedings are confidential, though an annual report to the authority to which the REC reports is required and must be available for public inspection[7] (p. 9). Again there seems to me no clear answer as to which is better — closed or open meetings. In favour of open meetings are that protection of the public is openly seen to be done, and that closed meetings tend to provoke suspicion in at least some members of any public used to democratic processes. In favour of closed meetings is that doubts and concerns and criticisms are for many, and especially perhaps for many health care professionals, more easily expressed, and thus more likely to be addressed, in closed meetings where the members know and trust each other.

National and local committees

Whether or not to have a national committee, whether or not to have local committees, must, it seems clear to me, be a matter for nations to decide for themselves. Again the underlying criteria for such decisions should be: which type of committee or combination of committees will best achieve the moral objectives of promoting beneficial medical research while protecting and respecting the subjects of that research?

Current 'permissive' CIOMS advice seems appropriate. It may however be worth proposing that for multi-centre research, for particularly controversial or potentially controversial research projects, and for new sorts of research on human subjects a national committee composed of 'exemplary' members, having both national standing and a high degree of the relevant types of expertise, might be very helpful in an advisory role. Their assessments would not be mandatory on other committees, but the clarity and scope of their arguments could be expected in many cases to reduce the need for extensive and time-consuming local review of the same issues.

Benefits and Harms

Non-therapeutic research

Two important principles of medical research seem worth enunciating explicitly. First, that in the case of non-therapeutic research, where there is no intention or prospect of benefiting the subject, only a minimal level of harm must be risked to the subject even if the benefits to others of the research are predicted to be extensive. The underlying assumption here is that the techniques of medicine are not to be used to impose more than a risk of minimal harm on a subject unless it is for the subject's own benefit. This is consistent with the spirit of the repeated theme of the Declaration of Helsinki that in medical research the interests of science and society should never take precedence over considerations related to the well-being of the subject, while allowing for volunteers to subject themselves to a low level of risk for the benefit of others. However, it remains a real problem to decide what sorts of levels of risk are acceptable, both in the context of true volunteers, where the subjects are autonomous, understand the issues and freely agree to participate, and in contexts where the subjects of non-therapeutic research are not autonomous, or not adequately autonomous (young children; severely mentally impaired subjects such as the severely mentally ill, severely mentally retarded and severely senile). So far as children are concerned it is now, I think, widely agreed in Britain, at least, that risks comparable to the ordinary risks of everyday life to which parents are permitted to expose their children for the benefit of others (for example, driving them in the family car in order to visit a lonely but unloved relative) are also acceptable in the context of non-therapeutic research on children; such was the conclusion of a British multidisciplinary working party[10] and I have recently argued in its favour, at greater length than is possible here.[11]

Non-therapeutic research and greater-than-minimal risk

If the subject is autonomous and volunteers to take greater than minimal risks for the benefit of others, is it ever justifiable to accept such an altruistic offer and carry out non-therapeutic research where the risk to the subject is greater than minimal (i.e., more than the risks of everyday life)? The British Royal College of Physicians, in its guidelines on research involving patients[12] (p. 11) envisages that such circumstances may, rarely, occur, and Dr Levine[9] (p. 46) indicates that his prime concern, along with that of the US National Commission Report,[13] is that subjects will have sufficient information to make their own informed decisions, provided any 'extreme case of unreasonable risk' has been excluded. While I find their arguments, based on respect for autonomy of the subject, attractive (it would be unacceptably paternalistic to prevent a subject who is autonomously prepared to undergo risky research in the altruistic service of others from doing so) I believe that the counter-arguments require a substantial control on the degree of risk to which research subjects should be allowed to agree to subject themselves for the benefit of others. These counter-arguments are, first, that the medical profession has a commitment to benefit and not to harm its patients — the Hippocratic commitment — and that that commitment is undermined by a readiness to impose, for the benefit of others, greater than minimal risks upon its research subjects. The autonomy of doctors individually and professionally to restrict the harm that they are prepared to do to others to harm that is intended for the harm-bearers' own benefit, should, I believe, be respected not only by members of the profession and their national and international representatives, but also by the societies in which doctors function. Helping their patients (and subjects) and not harming them (even for the benefit of others) is the sort of work to which doctors autonomously wish to commit themselves and they should be allowed to continue to do so. Acceptance of a minimal-risk level of harm as permissible in non-therapeutic research is already a modification of the original Helsinki principle, which if interpreted strictly would *never* allow imposition of *any* degree of risk for non-therapeutic purposes. The special trust of patients in doctors, and the special commitment of doctors to their patients, would, I believe, be seriously threatened by allowing doctors to subject even the most willing subjects to substantial risks for the benefit of others, which would be bad for both patients and doctors. It would be bad also for public policy — and here I offer a utilitarian, welfare-maximization argument, which claims that an erosion of public trust in doctors would damage the public welfare, not only by alarming patients in the ordinary therapeutic relationship but also, I suspect, by creating a public backlash against *any* sort of medical research, with ever more stringent legal restrictions being imposed to constrain it.

Two qualifications

Two qualifications, however, are needed of my own position. The first is that the *possibility* of greater than minimal-risk research being of such enormous benefit to others that it would be justifiable to accept volunteers should not be *absolutely* ruled out but left open for possible exceptional circumstances. The second qualification is that reasonably consistent standards for acceptable 'minimal risk' need to be established, probably by examples, and these standards should be related to similar levels of acceptable risk in everyday life. The Royal College of Physicians guidelines, for example, suggest that the risk of dying from flying as a passenger on a scheduled aircraft is an everyday risk that can reasonably be regarded as 'minimal' and that non-therapeutic research that produces that level of risk of dying is acceptable. But what about the risk of a nephrectomy? At present the medical profession allows a family member to volunteer to donate a kidney to another family member. Although this is not a risk borne in the context of medical research, it is a 'non-therapeutic' risk borne by a volunteer for the altruistic purpose of greatly benefiting another, a loved one, and imposed by a medical action. We need to try to integrate such cases into a coherent approach to the imposition of medical risks for the benefit of others.

Therapeutic research

Here the objective seems far clearer and better established. Risk to the subject is permissible insofar as it is justified by the prospect of a net medical benefit to that subject, which is the same justification as for any risk imposed by a doctor on a patient in the therapeutic relationship. This, of course, means that in some contexts the permissible risks of therapeutic research may be very much greater than the risks permissible in non-therapeutic research, but only where such risks are justified by the prospect of net medical benefit for the subject. As an example it is only necessary to recall the very considerable risks of many anti-cancer drugs. Their use in non-therapeutic research might well be forbidden because of those risks — but for patients with cancer the potential for net medical benefit of participation in a therapeutic trial of two anti-cancer agents may justify their use in therapeutic research.

Protocols should specify the intended benefits and the intended beneficiaries of the research as well as the anticipated risks and risk bearers

If there is agreement on these background assumptions concerning risk of harm and probability of benefit it seems to me that the CIOMS guidelines should specify briefly the content of the assumptions and include around them a section on the information required from researchers. In particular, questions about potential benefits and risks of projects should specifically address the questions of who the intended/expected beneficiaries are, the nature and extent of the various harms and benefits anticipated (including, if relevant, physical, psychological and social harms and benefits), and some assessment of their likelihood or probability. (The Royal College of Physicians guidelines give some indication of the interaction of extent and nature of harms with their probabilities — a small probability of a mild headache, for example, versus a 'very remote chance of serious injury or death', relating the latter, as stated above, to the risks of flying in scheduled aircraft[8] (p. 21).) Although information about risks is notoriously difficult to obtain, it seems reasonable to encourage researchers to try to do so, and to quantify such information, even if only roughly.

As the 1982 CIOMS Guidelines state, scientific validity must be established, directly or indirectly, by a REC, for if a project is not scientifically valid it cannot produce benefits, and then all risks of harm associated with it become morally unacceptable in that there can be no benefit to justify them. It may be that the taking of precautions against fraudulent presentation of results is similarly justifiable, quite independently of arguments rejecting fraud on grounds that deceit is intrinsically wrong.

Financial benefits

Self-interest is well known to distort people's judgement on behalf of others, to the likely detriment of those others. Therefore it is part of the duty of a REC to elicit the self-interest of researchers and their departments in promoting their projects. Hence routine inquiries are advisable about the financial benefits to researchers and their departments from carrying out particular projects, and the RCP guidelines[8] (p. 40) and the British Government guidelines[7] (p. 14) require that such payments be reported to the committee or (RCP) its chair or a sub-committee.

A concern about the moral problems that may be associated with payments should not be confused with the belief that payments are in themselves immoral. Problems arise only if the payments distort the judgement of researchers, members of ethics committees or subjects in a morally unacceptable way. Thus researchers *may* be induced to pay less scrupulous attention to the risks of an investigation if it is very greatly to their financial advantage that they carry it out; ethics committee members *may* be less critical of a project if they have been paid by the sponsoring organization; research subjects *may* be more inclined to volunteer *against their better judgement* if they are to be heavily rewarded for their participation than if they are to receive nothing except reimbursement of their actual expenses. In all cases the primary concern of RECs should be to elicit the nature and extent of any payments and then to make a judgement about whether or not the interests of the research subjects can be adequately protected in the context of those payments. In the particular case of payment to subjects it seems to me that there is a real danger of under-rewarding subjects on the mistaken basis that this somehow protects them. We should be concerned that subjects make adequately autonomous decisions in deciding whether or not to volunteer for research projects. The fact that they are paid does *not* show that they are *ipso facto* unable to make adequately autonomous decisions — and, if it did, then we had all better review our competence to make adequately autonomous decisions in contexts where we have been paid. The objective, perhaps, should be to avoid payments that are large enough to encourage people to make decisions that are contrary to their better judgment.

Permission to inform the subject's general practitioner

One important means of protecting research subjects is to confirm that their state of health is not such as to make participation particularly risky. Thus the British Government guidelines[7] (p. 12) require that RECs should establish that the researcher accepts responsibility for ascertaining whether subjects are medically fit to participate, obtains information about any current medication or treatment, and obtains permission to communicate where appropriate with the subject's general practitioner, refusal of such permission disqualifying potential subjects from being used as research subjects.

Compensation for harm caused by participation as a research subject

In the case of non-therapeutic research, or research that is in part non-therapeutic in its intent, there seems to be a very strong argument in favour of the researching organization undertaking to compensate any subject who is harmed by altruistic participation in research designed to benefit others[9,14] (pp. 117-123, 168-169). In this context there is, in my personal opinion, an unacceptable double standard in Britain whereby pharmaceutical companies provide (and are expected to provide) no-fault compensation for research subjects injured as a result of their participation, while the universities, the National Health Service and the government's Medical Research Council have no such obligation to the subjects of their research, though all three have a reasonably sympathetic system for *ex gratia* payments. The Royal College of Physicians guidelines urge that the existing situation be changed so that all healthy volunteers should be compensated for any ill-health or injury caused by their participation as research subjects, independently of proof of negligence; and the Medical Research Council in Britain has accepted the recommendation of the Medicines Commission that there should be advance assurance of adequate compensation without the need for the volunteer to show negligence[8] (pp. 33-39).

Nonetheless there is no legal or contractual right to such compensation where the research is carried out in the public sector, and the British Government guidelines[7] affirm that "NHS bodies are not empowered to offer advance indemnity to participants in research projects", and that volunteers "must therefore be told in advance of all known risks and be made aware that there could also be unforeseen risks, and of the possible difficulties in obtaining compensation" (p. 14). While this is undoubtedly autonomy-respecting, (a) it is likely to discourage participation in non-therapeutic research, and (b) it evades the question of moral responsibility for compensation, regardless of fault, if harm does arise. It seems clear that, if it is morally necessary to try to protect volunteer research subjects from harm, then it is also necessary for those responsible for inflicting any such harm that does arise to accept responsibility for reducing its adverse effects — and compensation is an important way of trying to reduce the adverse effects of a harm. I believe that the revised CIOMS guidelines could very usefully strengthen the 1982 guidelines on compensation by recommending pre-commitment by *all* bodies sponsoring non-therapeutic research, *including governmental bodies*, to compensate subjects for harm caused by such participation, where causation is established 'on the balance of probabilities', and whether or not negligence has occurred or been demonstrated. And, finally, the CIOMS epidemiology research guidelines[4] suggest that an expression of regret, and an apology if indicated, as well as reparation, may be important requirements if harm has resulted from research (p. 22-23).

Prior scrutiny of proposals by a senior clinician

One further protection for subjects recommended by the Royal College of Physicians report[8] (p. 14 and p. 12) is that research applications by junior staff or by those who do not bear ultimate clinical responsibility for research subjects should, before being sent to the REC, be scrutinized by a physician responsible for subjects' medical care, whether hospital consultant or general practitioner, who should assess 'the quality of both science and ethics'. This seems a beneficial and practical proposal.

Respect for Autonomy and Adequately Informed Consent

As argued above, to do things to people without giving them adequate information about what one proposes and why, and without their consent, is to infringe their autonomy. This fact about morality applies as much in therapeutic medicine as in non-therapeutic research, but given the Hippocratic assumption (that the doctor will only propose doing something if it is for the patient's medical benefit) patients may well be content (and of course often are) to accept the doctor's proposals with very little additional information in the case of therapy intended for their own (above all, for their own) benefit. In the case of non-therapeutic research the Hippocratic assumption does not apply and therefore the researcher has to be particularly scrupulous to make this clear to the subject, and to give him or her adequate information about what is proposed and why, including of course the hoped-for benefits for others, and what the risks of harm and even of mere inconvenience are. This process of giving adequate information and explanation, and seeking the subject's deliberated agreement and *permission* to proceed, is the process of obtaining (adequately) informed consent, and its moral purpose is respect for the patient's autonomy. Related concerns are non-deceit, respect for the patient's physical and mental and social 'integrity' (where any action that risks infringement of such integrity infringes the person's autonomy unless adequately informed consent to that action has been obtained), respect for the person's privacy (for similar reasons), and respect for the person's confidences (sometimes seen as an aspect of respect for privacy). These general principles are well established in contemporary guidelines to RECs, including the 1982 CIOMS guidelines. However perhaps the revised CIOMS guidelines should flesh out these general principles with examples from national guidelines. Thus, provision of an information sheet to subjects seems a highly desirable method of providing adequate information (with accompanying methods for explaining/translating it where necessary) in all but the most trivial-risk research. The more complicated the research, the more important for this information sheet to be written or at least revised by experts in communication with the public (e.g. popular journalists). An excellent example is the general information booklet about clinical trials[15] provided by the patient education group of the Royal Marsden Hospital, a leading British cancer hospital.

Research that involves both therapeutic and non-therapeutic intent

The polar examples of therapeutic and non-therapeutic research are easy to discern. A research project where there is no intention or reasonable prospect of medically benefiting the subject is non-therapeutic research; examples might be the testing of excretion-rates of new drugs, or the effects on healthy skin of a new topical medication, in healthy volunteers. A clear example of therapeutic research is a research project comparing two standard cancer therapies in which the researchers have no good reason to believe that one therapy is better than the other, where the intent is to provide maximal medical benefit for the patient subjects, and for which purpose the comparison is necessary and in the patient's interests. Of course, many clinical research projects combine both intentions: to provide maximal benefit for the patient subject, and to elicit generalizable knowledge that will benefit future patients.

80

I know of no way of quantifying the balance between therapeutic and non-therapeutic intent. Nonetheless, I believe an essential question for RECs to ask researchers and themselves is: to what extent is the intention of the proposed research to produce the best available medical benefits for the subjects (therapeutic research), and to what extent is it intended not for the benefit of the subjects but for the benefit of others (non-therapeutic research)? Expressed differently, how many procedures is the subject to undergo that would not have been necessary had the sole intention been to produce greatest available medical benefit for the patient with least harm or risk of harm for the patient, in all senses of harm, including disturbance and inconvenience? The more the project lies towards the non-therapeutic end of the spectrum, the more researchers should: (a) make explicit to subjects that the Hippocratic commitment is modified and that their participation for the sake of others as well as themselves is being solicited; (b) give subjects adequate information about the pros and cons of such participation; and (c) ensure that the risks anticipated for subjects are no greater than minimal.

Conversely, the more the research project lies towards the therapeutic end of the spectrum, the more the Hippocratic commitment applies (of doing to the patient only what the doctor believes will produce the best available net medical benefit for that patient) and the less appropriate therefore is it to require special approaches to information-giving and the obtaining of consent, over and above the normal requirements of therapeutic clinical practice. And in ordinary clinical practice, underpinned as it is by the Hippocratic commitment, the question of how much information to give the patient is primarily determined by how much information the patient wants to have; some patients want as much information and involvement in therapeutic decision-making as do subjects in non-therapeutic research, but many patients, especially those who are very sick, prefer to accept and trust in the Hippocratic commitment of the doctor to do his or her best for the patient, and to leave to the doctor decisions about their treatment, the amount of information to give them, and so on. The doctor is respecting the patient's autonomy just as much in respecting *those* preferences as in giving patients who want it the information they request and involving them in decision-making when this is what they prefer.

Thus *in clear cases of therapeutic research* I believe that RECs should rely heavily on the researching clinicians' assessments of the preferences of individual patients, and I agree[16] with Chalmers and Baum that a 'double standard' between ordinary clinical practice and research is morally inappropriate.[17] But a 'double standard' — i.e., a different standard — is entirely appropriate for non-therapeutic research, precisely because of the modification of the Hippocratic commitment, and researchers override subjects' autonomy in so far as they fail to inform their subjects about the non-therapeutic aspects of any research in which they intend to involve them.

Justice

As stated above, research ethics committees have not been set up to assess the distributive-justice or resource-allocation aspects of research projects. The guidelines should make this explicit.

As far as justice qua respect for morally acceptable laws is concerned, as the Royal College of Physicians guidelines[8] point out, "The public will reasonably expect that research involving human subjects is conducted in accordance with the law" (p. 18). In countries where legal systems are democratic and laws responsive to the will of the people, and doctors and other medical researchers committed to the welfare of patients, it is sometimes difficult to imagine that ethics committees should concern themselves explicitly either with concerns about the legality of research proposals ('of course, medical researchers would not propose to do anything that is illegal') or with concerns about the moral acceptability of laws relating to medical research. Nonetheless the lessons of history show that both assumptions can be wrong, and it therefore seems wise for the guidelines to require RECs to assure themselves both that research projects are legal according to the laws of their country and that the laws relating to medical research are morally acceptable. Neither requirement should be seen as providing significant new business for lawyers. The first requirement might involve a standard question to researchers requesting confirmation that the research proposed is lawful. Only in areas of significant doubt would legal advice be necessary. The second involves RECs assuring themselves that morally unacceptable research proposals are not being proposed on the basis of laws that are themselves morally unacceptable and that permit or even encourage such research on human subjects. Such issues would arise only if morally unacceptable research were being proposed that nonetheless conformed to the law. In such cases it would, I believe, be the duty of RECs not only to reject the research proposals but also to take such steps as are available to them — probably via their national medical bodies — to try to have the offending law that sanctions such research changed.

Finally, justice as respect for rights. Many current guidelines refer to the duty to protect research subjects' rights, as does the general survey (p. 4) preceding the 1982 CIOMS Guidelines, and I have no doubt that this is a proper objective. But which rights? Rights are essentially justified claims imposing positive or negative duties on others. One way of specifying the rights to be protected would be to try to list all the rights that research subjects have and to affirm or acknowledge them. Starting such a list would be doubtless fairly easy: the right not to have one's bodily, mental or social integrity infringed without one's adequately informed consent; the right not to be used as a research subject for the benefit of others without one's adequately informed consent; the right not to participate in research; the right to withdraw from participation in research; the right not to have one's medical care impaired by research; the right not to be unjustly excluded from participation in research. However, I suspect that completing the list would become an impossible task, especially in the CIOMS Guidelines, given their international audience. An alternative approach might be to affirm (a) that participation in medical research should never require subjects to abrogate or waive any of their existing rights, and (b) that all duties specified in the accepted research ethics guidelines of a jurisdiction can properly be acknowledged as also entailing the corresponding rights of research subjects. Thus research subjects would be acknowledged to have a right to be treated in accord with whatever guidelines were accepted in a particular jurisdiction, and the CIOMS guidelines would seek to inform the content of national guidelines. Thirdly, a subset of the duties described in a set of accepted guidelines could be designated as entailing corresponding rights in research subjects. One way or another, it seems to me that reference to subjects' rights in the 1982 CIOMS Guidelines (p. 4) ought to be clarified and made more specific.

Research Involving Special Classes of Research Subject

Although this is not strictly part of my brief, it does seem worth proposing that the moral 'specialness' of each group concerned should be made explicit. What are the moral features that account for special requirements in the assessment of the ethics of research on, for example, children, pregnant and nursing women, prisoners, mentally ill or retarded people, unconscious people, severely ill people, the vulnerable elderly, other especially vulnerable groups, colleagues and students and employees, and embryos and fetuses? At present both CIOMS guidelines and national guidelines tend to state differences in the ways research on such groups should be assessed, but do not make explicit the underlying moral rationale (which, I believe, can usually be readily made explicit in terms of extra obligations of researchers and RECs to protect those who are particularly vulnerable, or to avoid overriding the autonomy of those whose autonomy is either inadequate or at special risk of being inadequately respected or protected; and some would add the obligation of just or fair distribution of the benefits and burdens of participation in research as a further morally relevant factor in the case of certain special groups).

Practical Impediments

In brief, I believe that the main practical impediments are lack of time and lack of sufficient numbers of committee members with education in the basic elements of ethical analysis and of its application to proposals for human-subject research. To remedy these problems I would recommend (a) that committee membership be recognized by employing authorities as requiring of committee members, say, a day per month of (paid) time (or whatever the actual requirement is locally — I was struck by Dr Levine's assertion that he devoted 30 per cent of his professional effort to the research ethics committee he chaired[9] (p. 213)), with paid time and course fees for attendance at courses designed for REC members (this requirement would entail, of course, that there are such courses). In addition, perhaps CIOMS might consider creating a source-book for REC committee members, containing basic advice relevant to functions of RECs, including some basic readings. A further enterprise, perhaps leading to greater consistency in the practice of RECs, would be the collection of actual case analyses and decisions made by RECs, contributing to a type of case law or 'casuistry' of applications of general ethical principles to specific cases in medical research. Selection and publication by CIOMS of 'exemplary' case analyses and decisions, attempting to reflect a representative international selection of acceptable analyses and decisions, would further build towards an internationally consistent approach.

Capacity Building

I am not entirely certain that I understand the evocative concept of 'capacity building for ethical review in developing countries', which I have been asked to consider. But if I understand Professors Abdussalam and Osuntokun correctly in their paper on this issue in relation to epidemiology studies,[18] then the point is that very few developing countries can afford to pay to build and maintain institutions for health research of any sort, including research into appropriate ways of carrying out and maintaining ethical review of medical research. My response is that in relation to ethical review of research we are all — or at least most of us are — *de facto* members of developing countries, for very little national attention has been paid to capacity building for national ethical review in most countries. In this regard the CIOMS Guidelines would surely help if they recommended all nations to plan a national strategy for ethical review of medical research. The synoptic proposals in the preceding paragraph might constructively contribute to such development.

Review of Research with Foreign Sponsors

In their important contribution[18] to the CIOMS volume on ethics and epidemiology, Professors Abdussalam and Osuntokun warn of twin dangers — a sort of Scylla and Charybdis for international ethics. On the one hand, there is the danger of what they call 'ethical imperialism', with ethics committees in the developed world dictating to communities and research subjects in the developing world as to what is morally acceptable and what is not. On the other hand, there is too great a readiness to accept different standards in different communities, and to say, for instance, 'well we would call that sort of thing immoral in our culture, but they don't seem to mind it there, so let's do it' — the danger of moral relativism (Abdussalam and Osuntokun scathingly cite, and reject as 'sheer fallacy', the view that respect for individual autonomy might not be applicable in certain developing countries (p. 129)). For my own part it seems clear that, while the four Beauchamp and Childress prima facie principles plus attention to their scope of application do indeed afford a basic but *universal* moral commitment as well as a basic but universal moral language and framework for moral analysis, this fact in no way entails the end of intercultural moral differences! On the contrary, since one of the principles is respect for people's autonomy, and since it seems empirically indisputable that people's autonomous decisions are at least significantly influenced by their cultural environment, to the norms of which, on the whole, people are deeply committed, it will follow that people in different cultures will interpret these four principles differently and also will balance or otherwise prioritize them differently, and will have different views about their scope of application. Such cultural variation does not entail moral relativism (I recognize this needs more thorough argument than I am offering here), but may merely indicate that universal prima facie respect for people's autonomy requires *de facto* respect for cultural variations in moral decision. Thus, to avoid the Scylla of moral imperialism, a readiness to respect differences in interpretation of the common moral commitments amongst different cultures is required from all.

Nonetheless the common moral commitments require that transgression of any one of these prima facie principles can only be justified by pointing to the overriding application of one or more of the others, or to some relevant scope difference. Thus all members of the international moral community can expect an explanation and justification of any proposed or actual overriding of any one of these principles. Unless it can be justified by one or more of the other principles, or by some legitimate exclusion based on their scope of application, the behaviour stands condemned as immoral — and universally immoral. Thus may the Charybdis of moral relativism be avoided.

In between clear cases of respect for different but clearly morally acceptable choices, on the one hand, and rejection of clearly immoral choices, on the other, will lie a substantial grey area in which some will believe and argue that particular choices clearly are immoral, while others will believe and argue that though they transgress one or more of the prima facie moral principles nonetheless they are justified either by the overriding application of one or more of the other principles or by some legitimate exclusion based on the scope of application of the principle offended against. I have no formula for settling such debates. I hope more than believe that continuing discussion, argument, and attempts at persuasion by reasoned justification of the positions held will gradually reduce acceptance or excuse of clearly wrong, clearly immoral, positions as being in the legitimate grey area of morally acceptable disagreement.

In addition, practical systems must be devised for decision-making when irreconcilable moral differences remain. One such, in the context of research on human subjects organized by foreign sponsors, is that proposed by the 1982 CIOMS Guidelines, which require the approval of RECs in both the sponsoring country and the host country. Both RECs would use the same framework of moral analysis, but doing so from different cultural perspectives might well come to differing conclusions. Only if they agreed on a proposal, perhaps modified after discussion and argument between the RECs involved and the researchers, could it go ahead.

All these proposed arrangements are imperfect — in the field of practical ethics what else might one reasonably expect? They do, however, move international thinking forward along potentially mutually agreeable and morally defensible lines.

References

1. Beauchamp T., Childress J. *Principles of biomedical ethics (3rd ed.)*. New York, Oxford: Oxford University Press, 1989 (1st ed. 1979).
2. Gillon R. *Philosophical medical ethics*. Chichester: Wiley, 1986 (reprinted 1990, 1991, 1992).
3. Stanley J.M. (ed.). The Appleton consensus: suggested international guidelines for decisions to forgo medical treatment. First published in the *Journal of the Danish Medical Association*, 1989; 109: 1035-1046. Reprinted in *Journal of medical ethics*, 1989; 15: 129-136.
4. Council for International Organizations of Medical Sciences (CIOMS). *International guidelines for ethical review of epidemiological studies*. Geneva, CIOMS: 1991.
5. The Nuremberg Code (1947). Variously reprinted. e.g. in: Duncan A.S., Dunstan G.R., Welbourn R.B., eds. *The dictionary of medical ethics* (revised edition). London: Darton Longman and Todd, 1981; 130-132.
6. World Medical Association. *Declaration of Helsinki* (1964, amended 1975, 1983, 1989). Variously reprinted. e.g., in Reference 5, 132-135.
7. (British Government) Department of Health. *Local research ethics committees — Health Service Guidelines*. London: Department of Health, 1991. Ref. HSG (91) 5. (Available from Department of Health, Eileen House, 80-94 Newington Causeway, Elephant and Castle, London, SE1 6EF).
8. Royal College of Physicians. *Guidelines in the practice of ethics committees in medical research involving human subjects (2nd ed.)*. London: Royal College of Physicians of London, 1990.
9. (United States) Department of Health and Human Services — Rules and Regulations. Reprinted in: Levine R.J. *Ethics and regulation of clinical research*. Baltimore, Munich: Urban and Schwarzenberg, 1981; 259-273. US Government regulations cited were applicable in 1981, when Dr Levine's book was published. In 1991 a common Federal Policy for the Protection of Human Subjects (Federal

Regulation, Vol. 56, No. 117, 18 June 1991) was issued. This Policy is summarized in the paper, in this volume, by Kelly, Fluss and Gutteridge, *The regulation of research on human subjects: a decade of progress*, under United States of America.

10. Nicholson R.H. (ed.). *Medical research with children: ethics law and practice*. The report of an Institute of Medical Ethics working group on the ethics of clinical research investigations on children. Oxford: Oxford University Press, 1986.

11. Gillon R. Research on the vulnerable — an ethical overview. In: Brazier M., Lobjoit M. (eds). *Protecting the vulnerable — autonomy and consent in health care*. London: Routledge, 1991, 52-76.

12. Royal College of Physicians. *Research involving patients*. London: Royal College of Physicians of London, 1990.

13. *(United States) National Commission for protection of human subjects of biomedical and behavioural research, report and recommendations; institutional review boards*. Washington, DC: Department of Health Education and Welfare, 1978, 24-25. (DHEW publication number (OS) 78-0008).

14. Silverman W.A. *Human experimentation — a guided step into the unknown*. Oxford: Oxford University Press, 1985.

15. Patient education group, Royal Marsden Hospital. *Clinical trials — your questions answered*. London and Surrey: Royal Marsden Hospital, 1990. (Distributed by Haigh and Hochland Ltd, International University Booksellers, The Precinct Centre, Manchester MI3 9QA, England.)

16. Gillon R. Medical treatment, medical research and informed consent. *Journal of medical ethics*, 1989; 15: 3-5, 11.

17. Chalmers I., Baum M. Consent to randomised treatment [letter]. *Lancet*, 1982, ii: 1051.

18. Abdussalam M., Osuntokun B.O. Capacity building for ethical consideration of epidemiological studies: perspective of developing countries. In: Bankowski Z., Bryant J.H., Last J.M. (eds) *Ethics and epidemiology: International guidelines — proceedings of the XXVth CIOMS Conference*. Geneva: CIOMS, 1991, 126-136.

REPORT OF WORKING GROUP B: ETHICAL REVIEW PROCEDURES

Moderator: **M.A.M. de Wachter**
Rapporteur: **J. Miller**

Working Group B focused on ethical review procedures particularly for research in which the sponsors or investigators are from a developed (initiating) country and the research is to be conducted in a developing (host) country. In addition, it addressed topics ranging from the relationship of law and ethics in the Guidelines to sanctions for non-compliance with ethical standards of research. The report is structured according to the questions or items posed by the conference organizers.

1. *Focus on research in which the sponsors and/or investigators are from a developed nation (initiating country) and the research is to be done in a developing (host) country*
   The group addressed exclusively the ethical aspects of research initiated in a developed country and carried out in a host country, but noted that the concern with ethical procedures would also apply to research within a developed country with groups such as native peoples. The ethical review procedures should accord with the principles of the Declaration of Helsinki and should be applicable to a broad scope of health-science research interventions in human subjects. These included use of drugs, devices, vaccines, biologicals, DNA probes, experimental surgery, research with oncogenes and so forth. (Some classes of research may be explicitly exempt from full review.)

2. *Ethical standards no less exacting than they would be for research carried out within the initiating country*
   The group was unanimous that only research found ethical by independent, prospective review in both countries and in conformity with the laws of the host country could proceed. Review by a joint committee from the two countries was considered impractical and unnecessary on the basis of past experience. The independent ethics review should be carried out in both countries according to common ethical principles, but not necessarily according to identical procedures.

   The well-accepted guiding principles of autonomy, beneficence, non-maleficence and justice, developed in the Western world, may require reformulation in less individualistic countries with different religious traditions.

   Reflecting on the suggestion of more pragmatic, rather than idealistic, standards the group reaffirmed the importance of aiming at high standards as an ideal in both developed and developing countries. Procedures to apply common principles might be modified to accommodate the circumstances of many developing countries (e.g., illiteracy, paucity of scientists to serve on ethical committees). Exceptions should be viewed as acceptable for a limited and defined time during which the country would be expected to remedy the situation. The CIOMS Guidelines should qualify the principles appropriately in the discussion sections.

3. *Where should ethical review take place?*
Review procedures in the two countries may differ. In developed countries, with well-defined local ethical committees, detailed review would take place in the committee of the institution where the investigator is employed. Some countries may also review at the national level, but a two-layer review should not be required. In developing countries, where there are few independent, multidisciplinary committees for ethical review of research, such review is likely, for the present at least, to take place through special committees at the national level. The capacity for more systematic ethical review in developing countries must be encouraged and will likely develop in concert with emergence of a national capacity to conduct research and not just to collaborate in research. If a national committee alone reviews a protocol, one or more representatives from the site where the research is to be conducted must be involved. As noted in the response to question 1, ethical approval by both committees was deemed necessary for research to proceed.

During the discussion, the group reflected on the relationship of ethics and law in the Guidelines and agreed that the Guidelines should emphasize the ethical principles and allow for differences in legal status of ethical committees in different countries. Several lawyers suggested linking bioethics explicitly with human rights conventions by mention of Article 7 of the International Covenant on Civil and Political Rights. It was agreed that research ethics committees must have the authority to collect information they deem necessary to protect research subjects.

4. *Responsibilities for ethical review in the two countries*
While committees in the initiating and host countries must review both ethics and scientific merit in an integrated way, the group defined special responsibilities for ethics review for the committee in the developing country:
a) to assess those aspects, such as informed consent, coercive conditions and feasibility of the project, that depend on intimate knowledge of the site, the culture, the proposed collaborating researcher, the subjects and so on;
b) to determine the relevance of the research to the needs of the host country; and

89

c) to consider the motivation for the research and for its conduct in the host country;

and for the committee in the initiating country:

a) to assess in detail the scientific validity of the proposed research;
b) to ensure that research that would be unethical in the initiating country is not approved for implementation in any other country; and
c) to protect subjects from exploitation and to assure that there is a sound motivation for conduct of the research in the host country.

5. *Responsibility for evaluating scientific design by research ethical committees*

The working group agreed that scientific and ethical review must be integrated. Therefore, the responsibilities of the local or national research ethical committees include evaluation of scientific design. With regard to whether local review is suitable for multicentre trials, given the inevitable duplication of effort that would result, participants with experience in reviewing multi-centre-trial protocols recommended that countries define a mechanism for such review early in the development of their ethical review systems. Various models are possible. For example, Denmark has a double-string system where the regional committee reviews the protocol first and then sends it to the local committee, with resort to the central national committee should problems arise. The United States, England and Canada rely, with rare exceptions, on local committee review as essential to ensure that the research is appropriate in a given institution and to preserve local autonomy and responsibility. It was also suggested that repeated review by local committees might help to identify potential problems and modifications needed in the protocol.

Regardless of the review mechanism chosen, double-string (Denmark), regional (Norway) or local (US, Canada, UK), it was suggested that benefits might ensue from centralized pooling of data to monitor safety; auditing of ethics committee review in multicentre trials to identify idiosyncratic behaviour; sharing among review committees of their perceptions of scientific or ethical flaws that might be of generalizable value for others assessing the protocol. Such sharing was seen as a useful means to promote sensitization and training with respect to any research reviewed by more than one ethics committee, not necessarily only for multicentre trials. In the case of research initiated in developed countries and carried out in developing countries, this would be the rule. Further consideration was suggested of needs of developing countries with respect to review of multicentre trials.

6. *Conformity of externally sponsored research with national and community priorities within the host country*

Initially the group was for delegating responsibility and coordination of the research with the host country's priorities to the ethical committee in the host country. However, after discussion of the many difficulties in setting clear national priorities (in both developed and developing countries) and the political nature of many priorities, the group agreed that this should not be the responsibility of an ethical review committee. An ethical review committee was unlikely to be sufficiently informed of initial steps in planning the research and was unlikely to have the breadth of exposure to a country's many sectoral needs. Further, the ethical authority of the ethical review committee should not be diluted by efforts to weigh national relevance. Research may be of priority through providing training opportunities and facilities even if it does not directly address diseases in the country. Priority-setting was viewed as a government responsibility, perhaps through a ministry of health, a granting body or a research council.

The working group recommended that, instead of national priorities as a whole, an effective measure might be that a project be of net benefit to the country. Requiring a comprehensive definition of priorities by the host country was seen as unrealistic and onerous. One participant noted that if a developing country could define all its priorities it would already be developed. In relation to priorities, the group held that the ethical committee had a responsibility to ensure that the research was sound and conducted in a competent and ethical fashion and with sufficient follow-through to be of use. It would not, for example, be reasonable to conduct research where medical devices that required upkeep and training were introduced without such support.

7. *Provisions to assure competence of the scientific and ethical review committees to build their capacities and to assure their independence*

The working group recognized the need for committee composition that included many disciplines, lay members who could represent community values, ethicists/theologians, men and women. It endorsed the participation of patients in ethics committees in some instances, particularly for chronic diseases with self-support groups (e.g. haemophilia, diabetes, multiple sclerosis). It strongly agreed with rotation of membership to blend experience with openness to cultural and scientific evolution. It supported the importance of members preserving confidentiality of review. It also agreed that committee members must not have a direct interest in the research proposal or in the sponsors (or beneficiaries?) of that research; suggested the possibility of an observer on the review committee to safeguard the review process; and urged continuing review and follow-up progress reports.

Beyond these points, the group emphasized the key importance of increasing review competence in developing countries. It sought means to remedy the paucity in developing countries of personnel trained in science and in ethics, despite perceived rapid increases in scientific capacity in at least some developing countries and increased speed of dissemination of research results from developed to developing countries.

As a first step, it was suggested that CIOMS might make an inventory of training and exchange programmes of use to developing countries. Several such programmes were noted (on the part of such bodies as the Fogarty Center, World Health Organization, World Pathology Foundation, International Development Research Centre of Canada, Canadian International Development Agency and MATCH). The group recognized the problem of ensuring that trainees returned to the host country. Ethics should be an integral aspect of the scientific training. True collaborative partnership research between researchers in developed and developing countries was seen as another important avenue. The familiarity of the researcher in the developed country with ethical review was viewed as important.

Partnership and sponsorship of research should not be limited to tropical diseases. Many participants agreed that the statement "there is no valid alternative to the use of subjects from developing communities" should be softened to allow the Third World to participate as full partners in research, rather than as vulnerable and exploitable populations. However, one participant expressed concern about weakening this protection for potential Third World subjects.

As to independence of ethical review committees, the Working Group acknowledged the difficulty in ensuring this and arrived at no clear mechanisms to achieve it.

8. *International resource groups*
The working group accepted the desirability of international resource groups to assist in aspects of ethical review. It identified several: CIOMS, the WHO Global and Regional Advisory Committees for Health Research, and certain disease societies. One function suggested for an international resource group was monitoring of compliance with research protocol. Dispute resolution was rejected as a function of such international groups, as, in the view of the Working Group, approval of

research requires approval by committees in both developing and developed countries.

9. *Sanctions for non-compliance with ethical standards for research*
With regard to sanctions for non-compliance with ethical standards for research, the group generally urged that sanctions be used as a last resort. Control should be exerted preferably through communication, development of an atmosphere of mutual trust, training, sensitization, education and support to help develop the capacity and understanding for ethical conduct of research in investigators, ethical committees, institutions engaged in and sponsoring research, and others involved. In short, medical research ethics rested primarily upon high standards of ethical research, interpreted in practical means such as informed consent, and exercised by trustworthy individuals of good will. Policing functions could erode the critical foundations of trust and pose problems both within a country and especially between countries.

To prevent problems and to address them should they occur, the group recommended simple inquiries, clear channels of communication, central resources for advice, and educational opportunities as the first approach. A "hot line", the offer of a site visit to examine the process of ethical review, and workshops to exchange information among those involved in research ethics have proved effective in correcting and improving ethical standards. In this context, the group reiterated the critical role of integrated ethics and health science training for investigators and health-care providers. Ethics teaching in medical faculties was noted as a fundamental tool, a first step for developing familiarity with ethical concepts and vocabulary, even if the teachers must learn along with the students. However, the group stressed the importance of a multidisciplinary approach to the process of ethical deliberation and the need to teach ethics with this appreciation. The ethical committee as a whole had ethical authority, not any single expert. The group recommended that CIOMS consider development of an inventory on ethics teaching or perhaps even organizing a future Round Table, given the enormous growth of the field and the wealth of resources on team and other approaches.

Should sanctions be necessary, the group noted the possibility of non-publication of results from research conducted in an unethical way — perhaps the most effective sanction, honoured consistently by reputable medical journals; loss of financial support for research; loss of eligibility for research grants; loss of licence to practise medicine; and, last and perhaps most onerous, compulsory service on an ethics committee.

10. *Information to be provided by investigators to ethical review committees*

The group identified a number of items that investigators should provide such as: how results will be forwarded to research subjects (not if), and financial arrangements. They should provide also a copy of the patient's information sheet and consent information to be conveyed, particularly for lay committee-members; information on any routine treatment that will be withheld from research subjects; special information intended for vulnerable subjects; details of insurance and compensation arrangements; the process to be used to communicate factors that affect harm/benefits; and regular progress reports.

11. *Embryo and fetal research, fetal tissue research, and genetics research*

Of these, genetic research was seen as the most significant for developing countries, likely to grow with the Human Genome Project and hence of high priority. Special note was made of the need to consider germ-line therapy, policies for DNA banks, consent, confidentiality, and definition of subjects in genetic and other familial-based research.

OBLIGATIONS OF SPONSORS

OBLIGATIONS OF SPONSORS:
A DEVELOPING-COMMUNITY PERSPECTIVE

E.N. Ngugi*

Introduction

Research involving human subjects is vital for the continued development of the individual, the family, the community and the entire human race. It must be a guiding principle of research workers to respect the dignity and self-determination of research subjects, recognizing their struggle to survive or just to be somebody. Subjects must be assured that the confidentiality of the information they share with the research worker will be safeguarded, that the researcher will be honest and upright with them, even in the event of failure or loss of face; this will earn the researcher respect and acceptance. The researcher must respect the right of the research subjects to be themselves and to enjoy basic human rights, including health services, within their social, cultural and economic structure.

It is therefore a responsibility of the sponsor to use a well-tested means of monitoring the research and to intervene if the rights or expectations of subjects are not being met.

To be an advocate of these principles a researcher must have synthesized them within his own values, thus avoiding any conflict with the meaning of life, living and interaction with research. The sponsor should be satisfied that the researcher has this philosophy, for this is what gives the researcher credibility.

This paper discusses the obligations of sponsors of research initiated in developed countries and carried out in developing (host) countries, in respect of four main areas:

1) Ensuring access of research subjects to research-related medical services;

2) Access to beneficial results of research;

3) Care and compensation for injury resulting from research;

4) Building up the capacity for research in developing countries.

Ensuring that research subjects have access to research-related medical services

Even in developed as well as developing countries, standards of quality of health care vary greatly, owing to lack or unequal distribution of resources and sometimes attitudes of providers and even users of health-care services. National and community health facilities may be inadequate. Hospitals may be so overcrowded that patients have to

* Department of Community Health, University of Nairobi, Nairobi, Kenya.

share beds, and thus transmit communicable diseases to each other. Outpatient departments are overcrowded with patients with controllable diseases. In such circumstances both the quality and the quantity of health care are affected. For instance, patients get minimal time — outpatients an average of only three minutes.

For research involving human subjects the researcher should be familiar with the resources available to the study population, and devise a strategy that meets both the research and the health needs of the study population. To establish a referral system may be one way of enabling those who need health care, other than that which is part of a study, to obtain such care, and also not to lose status or be discriminated against in any way because of participation in the research. Equally important, research subjects should not be required to attend for health care at facilities they would not choose to attend. Also, the facilities that research subjects attend should not be given unacceptable descriptive names: this will avoid subjects being victimized by employers, fellow workers or other people.

Sponsors must consider the funds they provide for recurrent expenditure on drugs, equipment and other health-care needs, so as to avoid an undue contrast between the health-care services provided under the auspices of the research project and the normal health-care services. It is questionable whether it is ethical to sponsor research that will cause a substantial imbalance in this respect, with no thought for the future. This risk may be reduced to a manageable level, particularly in the case of operational research, if a sustainability mechanism is built into the research project. Otherwise, the sponsor may disturb a coping mechanism that people may find difficult to restore when the study has ended.

The third consideration is that of health personnel, their potential and limitations, both administrative and clinical. Sponsors should be aware of staffing norms and appreciate the reasons for what may be considered inadequate norms; this is a useful indicator of the role that local professionals can play as well as their individual and collective responsibility. The research proposal should specify this and it is the sponsor's responsibility to ensure that the monitoring system can pinpoint gaps and weaknesses and to direct the project accordingly.

Access to beneficial results of research

It should be a sponsor's prime duty to ensure that the study subjects are among the first, if not the first, to profit from the outcome of a research project, whether it is a HIV or malaria vaccine or a female condom. Only subjects would suffer any unintended harmful outcome of the research, particularly physical or psychological harm; and notwithstanding the assistance which the system may provide, it is only the individual who can truly experience the pain and discomfort or other adverse physical or mental effects of the research procedure. The pain of the body is inseparable from that of the mind.[1]

To amplify this point: having access to, for example, treatment for gonorrhoea by a single dose of a drug that is 98-100% effective should be considered not a privilege but a right. Sponsors should discourage research that would benefit the developed sponsoring nation more than the developing host country, which provided the study subjects for the research.

It cannot be ethical to continue to use developing countries for research purposes merely because it is only those countries that can ensure the right study population, the lowest costs and the right environment. It is well appreciated that one of the reasons given, for example, for not making beneficial results of drug trials available is that drugs are expensive. It should be for the sponsor to bridge the gap by making sure that research subjects benefit from the result. If they cannot afford the drugs or the services, they should be given them free of charge, as far as possible, or at a price they can afford.

The proposal should state clearly how the research outcome will benefit the research subjects, and they should be informed of this before the study begins. Also, as a matter of principle, they should be consulted as to their expectations, and both parties should agree on what is realistic to achieve. All in all, there should be a fair distribution of benefits.

It is important also that the study population be told of the research findings and, from time to time, how the results are being used for the benefit of mankind locally, nationally or globally. In other words, they should share the sense of having accomplished something worthwhile, thus cementing their partnership with the investigators.

There should be written guidelines on how information will be shared with the subjects. To aid in doing so, the sponsor will make sure that the research proposal has been approved by the country's ethical committee and other pertinent bodies, and especially by the study subjects.

Care and compensation for injury resulting from research

Accidental injury to subjects of clinical or biomedical research, and resulting in temporary or permanent disability or even death, though extremely rare, can happen.[2] Subjects who suffer such injury, or their parents or guardians, should be informed of the nature and consequences of the injury and of the short-, medium-, and long-term prognosis, and counselled honestly and without prejudice. Definite arrangements should be made to respond appropriately. The sponsor ensures that the subject is not deprived of health care or socioeconomic support because of bias arising from racial, social, cultural or economic factors or associated with gender, age or imprisonment. A country's worker-compensation regulations will indicate how workers are compensated for different types of occupational injury and disability.

The complex issue of pregnancy and unsatisfactory outcome associated with research needs special attention to the circumstances of the pregnancy and the effects of an unsatisfactory outcome on the parents or the single mother. In case of death due to a research procedure the subject's next of kin should be identified and compensation paid in full and without delay.

Building up a developing country's research capacity

The sponsor must judge whether, or the extent to which, the country's prospects for developing research capacity are realistic, and whether nationals are motivated to carry out research or they are near the "burn-out" stage from overwork and poor pay. It is the sponsor's role to assess or recognize the country's potential and to help in consolidating and realising it. The responsible nationals are much better placed than outsiders to assess sociocultural barriers and political climate, and to decide which administrative structure could best assure development and implementation of research, and subsequent sustainability. To this end the sponsor should assure "on-the-job" training as well as support training specifically in research. For on-the-job training the co-researchers/trainers must be experienced and skilled in research methods and ready to share their expertise systematically, thus establishing a partnership with the host-country's researchers. They will also learn from their counterparts.

One aspect of research capability in particular need of support is the analysis and reporting of data. Too often, data collected in a developing country must be analysed in a developed country; the developing country may even be the last to learn about the findings. The sponsor should see that the investigator indicates in the research proposal how the data are to be analysed, what data-analysis facilities exist locally, how it is proposed to make available the necessary materials and equipment, such as a computer, in the host country, and whether national data-analysts have been identified and trained.

The sponsor should know of the host country's research capability, and whether the country's manpower development policy provides for training health personnel in research methods in their basic or continuing education.

Other crucial aspects of research capability are laboratory facilities and the necessary trained personnel, and the possibility of being well-informed about, as well as disseminating, research findings. When the host country is a developing country it should be given priority in being informed of the findings of the research which it hosted, and in applying them in health care. The sponsoring body will thus have fulfilled its obligations to human welfare, and the researcher to the observance of ethical principles.

In conclusion, the sponsor must understand the design of the proposed research, including the criteria for selecting research subjects, and be satisfied that the objectives and methods do not conflict in any way with basic human rights.

References

1. Ngugi E.N. 1977, Nursing Management of Pain, *Kenya Nursing Journal*.
2. Council for International Organizations of Medical Sciences, 1982, *Proposed International Guidelines for Biomedical Research Involving Human Subjects*, Geneva, CIOMS.

OBLIGATIONS OF SPONSORS: A SPONSORS' PERSPECTIVE

N.P. Maurice*

Introduction

To set the current scene this paper reviews the evolution of international drug development standards over the last decade. This is followed by an outline of a pharmaceutical industry viewpoint of its obligations when sponsoring human research, which should serve as a basis for the revision of the Proposed Guidelines.

(*Note*: For this paper a sponsor is a pharmaceutical company as opposed to an academic institution or clinician performing independent research, and the pharmaceutical industry, or industry, refers to the larger multi-national sponsors unless otherwise stated.)

Setting the Scene

When the original CIOMS Proposed Guidelines for Biomedical Research involving Human Subjects were being developed, activities with a similar goal were being followed by the United States Food and Drug Administration (FDA). The similarity in the goals of the two endeavours was in their desire to inhibit the deliberate or unwitting exploitation of underprivileged and other special populations, by enhancing the awareness of human rights and the need to fully respect them. In the decade since the introduction of these two codes of conduct a pharmaceutical "industrial revolution" in the conduct of industry-sponsored human research has occurred. Generally known as "Good Clinical Practice" (GCP), the revolution was primarily triggered by the FDAs human rights requirements becoming law in 1980/81, and has been given further impetus by the European Economic Community's Note for Guidance "On Good Clinical Practice for Trials on Medicinal Products in the European Community", which became operational in July 1991. In several additional countries, e.g., Australia, Canada, India, and Japan, government or industry has introduced, or is developing, a national GCP.

What is GCP?

As already indicated, GCP is a code of conduct for clinical research. Based on the Declaration of Helsinki, it provides detailed guidance/directions on the obligations of sponsors, investigators, ethics committees and regulatory authorities, in order to protect the integrity/rights of trial subjects. It requires sponsors to employ appro-

* Corporate Human Research Quality Assurance, Ciba-Geigy, Basel, Switzerland.

priately qualified and trained personnel. Also it requires them to use written standard procedures/instructions (standard operating procedures (SOP)) to enhance the performance and adequately document clinical research activities to be able to verify that the research has been performed according to GCP. Although the GCPs are generally intended for drug development research, one of them, that of the EEC, requires GCP also to be applied to *post-registration phase-IV trials.* Compliance with GCP needs to be confirmed through audits/ inspections performed by the regulatory authorities; but to date these have been systematically implemented only by the FDA.

How has GCP revolutionized clinical research?

With ever-increasing momentum the industry has recognized the need to perform research according to an established form of GCP. This has resulted in the general intention to apply GCP to all clinical trials in all phases and in all countries, even in those countries with no GCP requirements. This approach is necessary because ethically the industry can not justify, internally or externally, the use of more than one standard for clinical research.

How does the GCP revolution
affect clinical research in the developing countries?

The impact of adopting one basic standard for clinical research is leading to the disappearance of the so-called exploitation of developing countries. It also confronts clinical research with new challenges to be overcome because the GCPs have been drawn up in and for developed countries. These challenges are thus due mainly to differences in the health-care traditions and systems, and in the cultures, of the developing country communities, rather than to pharmacogenetic differences.

Other factors influencing the revolution

As already stated, only the EEC GCP applies to post-registration trials. However, in reality it must be realized that in the 1990s there will be no more trials that are not for regulatory use. This is for four main reasons:

1. More and more, regulatory authorities require "safety updates" on a drug when they review a registration application or at intervals after approval. This must include clinical-research safety data as well as spontaneous reports.

2. There is an increasing demand that registration applications include information on ongoing and planned trials. This can result in a demand for information on outcome when the application is reviewed, which frequently occurs only one to two years after the clinical dossier is written.

3. Phase IV trials frequently generate new information within the approved framework of a drug. This new information may be needed to modify the claims or for promotional purposes. Here again the regulatory authorities become involved.

4. The periodic revalidation of approved drugs is also becoming a standard requirement of the regulatory authorities. Trials performed since approval can be critical in sustaining the approved status.

Clearly the performance of trials in such a way that they will not be accepted by the regulatory authorities must be regarded as unethical and will lead to their disappearance. The above-mentioned factors, together with the increasing international linking of regulatory authority communications, are:

— accelerating the application of GCP to all phases of clinical research;

— leading to the disappearance of "marketing support" or "seeding" pseudo-trials;

— stimulating the introduction of post-marketing surveillance (PMS), prospective cohort studies aimed at generating more reliable information on the safety profile of drugs. These studies do not fall under GCP; indeed in Japan where they were formally implemented in July 1991 the activity runs under the title of Good Post-Marketing Surveillance Practice (GPMSP).

Since 1989 a concerted effort has been developing between the regulatory authorities and industry associations in the three major areas of drug development, the EEC, the USA and Japan. The objective of this group is to achieve the international harmonization of drug development, and the Nordic Council and the World Health Organization were involved in the First International Conference on Harmonization, in November 1991.

All these changes are also contributing to ensuring that human research is performed uniformly according to one global standard.

Finally, it must be noted that WHO has publicized the fact that it is also considering the need for a WHO GCP, but it is suggested that the revision of the "Proposed Guidelines" could serve that purpose. The matter could be resolved simply by changing the title of the document, for, in the opinion of the pharmaceutical industry the issue of two similar documents through WHO could prove to be more confusing than beneficial and should be avoided.

Obligations of Sponsors

The ethical obligations of sponsors of human research are manifold (hereafter referred to as the Obligations). They are dictated primarily by the current version of the Declaration of Helsinki (Hong Kong 1989), an established national or regional form of GCP, and other national requirements (when more demanding than the sponsors' standard). The Obligations are best reviewed by considering how each stage of the clinical research process and the people involved in that stage are affected when the research is conducted to meet those Obligations.

The stages of clinical research are:

1. Preparation;
2. Performance;
3. Evaluation, reporting and close-out;
4. Consequences.

The people involved are:

1. Sponsor's team;
2. Investigator and his/her team;
3. Ethics review body;
4. Regulatory authority representatives;
5. Trial subjects;
6. Societies (communities) affected by the research.

Basic obligations of sponsors

Before embarking on a review of the sponsors' obligations, attention must be drawn to the fundamental obligation that at every stage of clinical research the maintenance of the integrity of trial subjects must be placed above all other considerations by all the people involved.

Sponsors have four additional basic obligations, which apply to every aspect of pharmaceutical research and development (R&D):

— the people (personnel) performing the research must be suitably qualified and trained for the tasks for which they are responsible;

— written standards must exist describing how to perform tasks, i.e., standard operating procedures;

— the assurance that obligations are being met must be provided by means of in-process quality control and independent audits, i.e., quality assurance;

— the relevant research and development documentation and data on a drug must be archived/stored in such a way that it is readily retrievable by the sponsor for a reasonable period. This is generally at least for the "lifetime" of the drug in question.

The knowledge that the previously described basic obligations are complied with in the preclinical development of a drug provides the assurance that decisions regarding human research are based on reliable data.

This is of great importance for assessing the benefits-risks factors when planning clinical research, i.e., the classical ethical *beneficence and non-maleficence* aspects.

Failure to meet an obligation may put a trial subject at risk or jeopardize a trial or indeed the outcome of the whole clinical research programme. In the latter two instances this could put tens or hundreds of trial subjects at unnecessary risk, and delay the regulatory approval and thus the availability of a product to the patient.

The detailed stage-by-stage obligations of sponsors

The first stage: Preparing for research

Obligations to be covered by the sponsor when preparing the initiation of a research project may be divided into company internal and external:

Internal

— Define the therapeutic advantage.

— Determine the target disease prevalence and geographical distribution (orphan drugs).

— Confirm the integrity of the clinical research programme (approvability).

— Allocate the resources necessary for the efficient execution of the programme/trial-related activities.

— Confirm the integrity of the individual trial (protocol) and its (justify, methodology) congruity with the case report form (CRF).

— Ensure adequate compensation/treatment for subjects in the event of trial-related injury or death and appropriate investigator indemnity.

— Ensure that sufficient trial-drug supplies will be available, prepared according to GMP.

— Ensure appropriate data processing/handling, analysis and reporting as appropriate.

— Ensure the safe archiving of the trial documents.

External

— Select qualified and experienced investigator centres (people and facilities) and ensure their availability (and that of suitable patients) for the trial period.

— Provide all relevant drug information to investigator (brochure).

— Mutually agree on (sign) the trial protocol and case report form (legal agreement).

— Ensure appropriate patient information and consent documents and procedures (cultural differences).

— Ensure the availability of a properly constituted independent ethics committee, and then (generally via the investigator) the review and acceptance of the proposed trial and documents *prior to* trial initiation.

— Ensure that the trial drugs can be safely stored, correctly dispensed, accounted for and disposed of (drug accountability).

— Reach agreement on sponsor (and regulator) source data verification and possible audits.

— Ensure that all the involved personnel at the investigator centre understand and agree to their roles in the trial, and those of the sponsor's team.

— Agree with the investigator on the procedures and distribution of responsibilities for data processing, analysis, and the reporting/publishing of the findings.

The second stage: Performing the trial

When the preparations have been completed the trial can commence. The main obligations, but by no means all, are then related to the monitoring activities. These monitoring activities consist primarily of checks to confirm that the sponsor and investigator-centre resources and activities required for the efficient completion of the trial according to the protocol continue to be available and to be performed as agreed on during the preparation stage. Activities not mentioned above under "preparation" are:

Internal

— None.

External

— Ensure the timely collection, assessment and reporting of serious adverse drug reactions.

— Ensure that investigators, ethics committees, regulatory authorities and trial subjects are promptly informed of new findings (non-clinical or clinical) likely to increase the risk to the subjects and/or affect the outcome of the trial.

- Check (confirm) the agreement of the data entered in the CRFs with the source data.

- Ensure the correctly signed completion and correction (cleaning) of CRF data entries.

- Check (confirm) the safe and correct dispensing and accounting of trial drug supplies, and of trial subject treatment compliance where appropriate.

- Conclude the trial only when no further data are required from the investigator, and the remaining trial supplies have been disposed of as agreed in the protocol.

The third stage: Evaluation, reporting and close-out

As intimated earlier, these activities may be performed internally or externally, so no differentiation will be made between the activity sites in this section.

- A report/publication must be prepared on every trial, whether concluded as planned or not.

- A report must address all assessments proposed in the protocol.

- The sponsor must ensure that the trial data are evaluated and reported, both statistically and medically, by appropriately qualified people.

- Reports/publications on clinical trials must be distributed to interested parties as required.

- When no further data-handling or publication is anticipated a trial is closed-out and the trial data must be archived in a rapidly retrievable way.

The fourth stage: Consequences

The information generated by a trial or a clinical research programme should result in recommendations which a sponsor should be willing to adopt. It is usually possible to identify a number of possible outcomes of clinical research activities already at the planning stage. The outcomes may be critical for decisions regarding the further development or intention to market a new product or to make new claims or restrictions on the use of marketed drugs.

Based on the outcomes, a decision-tree can be drawn up of the ways in which a sponsor could respond to the foreseeable outcomes. Today sponsors should consider the outcomes and the responses which they would be willing to adopt. The body that functions as the sponsor's medical-ethical conscience should then be asked to determine whether it is justifiable to initiate the activity or not. Their decision should be binding. The sponsor should be organized to react to the outcome of a trial/programme without undue delay. The duty-of-care aspects should also be in the foreground and the risks and benefits to patients or potential patients carefully considered.

Conclusion

The marked changes that have occurred over the last decade in the way in which the industry performs human research are leading to a global implementation by the pharmaceutical industry of a single standard primarily based on the Good Clinical Practice code of conduct.

Whilst the adoption of a single standard is resulting in the disappearance of so-called "exploitationary" clinical research practices in the developing countries, it is introducing new challenges in the need to find acceptable ways of implementing GCP in countries with different health care traditions and different cultures. These challenges need to be overcome by the implementation of practical solutions jointly developed by the industry, academic medicine and the regulatory authorities. In the meantime achievement of this goal will be furthered by the introduction of the revised edition of the CIOMS Guidelines. These will undoubtedly give the necessary guidance to developing countries and subsequently provide support for the internationally acceptable form of GCP which will emerge from the international harmonization activities.

REPORT OF WORKING GROUP C: OBLIGATIONS OF SPONSORS

Moderator: **R. Gillon**
Rapporteurs: **W. Mariner** and **M. Abdussalam**

Group C was asked to consider the ethical obligations of sponsors and investigators from a developed country (as external sponsors) in research to be conducted in a developing (host) country.

Two threshold problems were identified but put aside as requiring more extensive analysis than permitted by the time available:

1. Whether focusing on externally sponsored research from developed countries to be conducted in developing countries adequately accounted for the range of circumstances in which ethical research required special attention to the concerns of people who suffer disadvantage or lack of resources, or are in other respects vulnerable or exploitable.

   The group concluded that it did not, and that the focus was arbitrary, because some people in developed countries had similar characteristics.

2. Whether externally sponsored research in developing host countries should be the subject of special ethical guidelines in addition to the general principles.

   It was concluded that, ideally, it should not. Nonetheless, the group proceeded to identify applications of the guidelines to clarify the general obligations of external sponsors.

Among the more general conclusions concerning the obligations of sponsors were the following (rationales omitted):

1. Research subjects and their communities should not be made worse off as a result of the research (apart from the justifiable risks of the research intervention), such as by the diversion of scarce resources.

2. Sponsors should be required to employ or train local investigators and personnel from the host country for the conduct of the research.

3. Sponsors should be required to provide financial, educational and other assistance for the development of independent scientific and ethical review committees in the host country. The funds should be provided to create or support an independent research infrastructure. To avoid any conflict of interest and to assure the review committee's independence, sponsors should provide funds to the host country government or research institution, and not directly to any review committee.

4. Sponsors and investigators should be required to provide or arrange for, or refer subjects for, health care for medical problems arising during the research. However, there should be no obligation to directly provide health care facilities over and above those necessary for the research. The provision of such facilities, and leaving them (and research equipment) with the country after the research, is to be encouraged as morally virtuous but not required.

5. On the question whether successful products of research, such as drugs, devices, etc., should be made reasonably available to the research subjects after such products have been developed, majority and minority positions were taken:

   Majority position: The majority's position was most ably articulated by those most familiar with the pharmaceutical industry. In this view, it is desirable but not ethically obligatory to provide access to the fruits of research to the research subjects and the host country as a first priority. One normative reason for this conclusion was that research subjects in developing countries are not entitled to a reward (for participating in research) that is not morally required for other research subjects. A second normative reason (with empirical underpinnings) is that if the resulting product or other benefit is scarce (i.e., if it is not feasible to produce a sufficient supply to meet all needs) the product ought to be made available first to those most in need of it. A third, quasi-normative, reason was that sponsors should not be discouraged from conducting research in cheaper places. Finally, a practical reason was that some elements of product distribution may be beyond a sponsor's control, such as a host country's requirement for drug registration/licensure, and sponsors should not be held accountable for obstacles beyond their control.

   Minority position: The minority questioned the normative claims of the majority position and argued that research in a developing country could be unjustifiable where no benefit was provided to the research subjects. In addition, any obligations of the sponsor could be made conditional on factors within the sponsor's control.

   Given the difficulty engendered by this issue, it should be considered by the Conference.

6. The group did agree that the sponsor be required to specify what, if any, resources, facilities, assistance and other "benefits" would and would not be made available to the research subjects and the host country during and after the research. This information must be included in the protocol and made clear before the study is approved. These specifics and the final details of the study should be agreed upon between the sponsor and the host country/

institution and other interested parties, including where relevant the community from which subjects are to be drawn. Such information must also be provided to subjects as part of the informed consent process.

7. The sponsors/investigators have an obligation to disclose to the proper authorities in the host country information that they discover from the study and is relevant to the health of the country or community.

8. It is justifiable to reimburse subjects for expenses or to pay subjects for their time and inconvenience occasioned by the conduct of research insofar as such payments do not override the subject's better judgment as to whether or not to participate in the research. Justifiable amounts were thought best determined specifically for each subject population, as long as they were not so high as to override judgment.

9. The group endorsed the concept that the sponsor has an obligation to provide compensation for injury to subjects arising out of participation in the research. "Injury" should be described as "not limited to physical injury" in order to indicate that psychological and social injuries (e.g., disclosure of confidential information) are included. It would be unwise to attempt to list specific kinds of injury owing to the risk of omitting any relevant category of injury. Also, the sponsor should pay the compensation to the subject expeditiously. (In cases in which another party might be responsible for the injury, the sponsor may be entitled to claim reimbursement or indemnification.)

10. Subjects should be informed of the availability and nature of compensation as part of the informed consent process.

11. Sanctions should be imposed on those who do not comply with the ethical principles of research. Although ethical review committees have no authority to impose sanctions, when such violations come to their attention they have a responsibility to notify the appropriate authorities who are so authorized. A system of sanctions for non-compliance should be established. Sanctions may include (a) refusal by licensing authorities to license/register licensable products resulting from the research, (b) the exclusion of such products from lists of approved or recommended products, such as WHO's list of approved drugs, (c) refusal to publish papers concerning the research, (d) the suspension or termination of the medical or professional licensures of those involved in misconduct, and (e) the termination of employment of, or of payments or other benefits to, individuals involved in misconduct.

The group also considered several more detailed issues of conducting research. It was agreed:

12. In multi-centre research, efforts should be made to minimize delays and disagreements occasioned by review by multiple review committees.

13. Ethics committees should require that sponsors/investigators of research involving drugs, vaccines, diagnostics and devices comply with Good Clinical Practices or equivalent standards governing manufacturing and distribution, and the qualifications and performance of sponsors and investigators. Similar standards of practice should be required for other kinds of research procedures and practices.

14. To avoid misunderstanding on the part of people invited to participate in market research and sales promotion studies, such studies should be clearly distinguished from clinical research and post-marketing research. Ethical review committees should reject from consideration market research, sales promotion studies, and post-marketing surveillance reporting.

15. Phase I drug studies or Phase I and II vaccine studies could be conducted outside the initiating or sponsoring country in developing host countries when the disease at issue occurs in both the sponsoring and the host countries.

16. It would be too restrictive to preclude research in developing communities unless there was no alternative to using such communities. Provided that a developing community has the disease and all other ethical principles and safeguards are satisfied, it would be acceptable to use that community. An example would be research to develop symptomatic relief of a condition existing in both developed and developing countries or communities, such as the common cold. This would permit research to be conducted where it was least expensive to do so.

17. The requirement that any individual's refusal to participate be respected should be modified to add an assurance that, where community leaders are involved in discussing or explaining the research, they actually represent the interests of the individual members of the community.

18. It would be inconsistent with respect for a person's refusal to participate in research to accept the consent of a community leader in the situation in which individual members of a community do not have the necessary awareness of the implications of participation in an experiment to give adequate informed consent directly to the investigators.

ETHICAL IMPLICATIONS OF STUDIES IN MOLECULAR GENETICS: AN EMERGING ISSUE

A.M. Capron*

Introduction: the scope of this essay

There is much that could be said about the implications of molecular genetics research for the protection of human subjects. As I describe briefly below, the field of molecular genetics is one of the most active in biomedical science today.[1] It has already produced useful drugs and biologicals, and further research on genetic methods for direct diagnosis and treatment of disease is proceeding rapidly and on many fronts. The purpose of this paper is not, however, to survey all aspects of molecular genetics as applied to human illness or even to discuss every possible implication for the regulation of research involving human subjects. Instead, I shall focus on the question: What aspects of molecular genetic research, if any, deserve special attention in the formulation of international guidelines for the ethical conduct of biomedical research involving human subjects? Specifically, I shall discuss the implications I see in various types of genetic studies for several of the Guidelines in the draft 1992 revision of the CIOMS Proposed International Guidelines.

My basic conclusion is that genetic research does not need to be treated separately in the Guidelines. Although it is a dynamic area of research in which powerful molecular tools are being developed, it is not unique. Special concerns also attend other cutting-edge areas of biomedicine, such as neuroscience and reproductive technologies. Most of the points raised in this essay can be accommodated through appropriate commentary under the existing Guidelines. Only in the case of germ-line genetic engineering are considerations presented that may not be adequately addressed by the proposed guidelines, and in many ways those points involve the ends of the research more than the means, whereas guidelines on research have typically been limited to ensuring the ethical acceptability of means, not ends.

Genetics research

Molecular genetic knowledge is relevant to research on human illness in the three classical activities of medicine: diagnosis, prevention and treatment. In addition to innovations in these three areas, studies of human beings are also carried out to gain the underlying molecular knowledge about human genes.

With the development of recombinant DNA methods in the mid-1970s the field of genetics began to enlarge markedly. Medical genetics

---

* The Law Center, University of Southern California, Los Angeles, California, U.S.A.

— a small discipline, often attached to pediatrics — had already begun to change, thanks to the development of biochemical methods of prenatal diagnosis. With the greater precision offered by molecular methods, knowledge about human genetics grew rapidly in quantity and precision. Indeed, the number of conditions listed in McKusick's catalogue of genetic diseases has grown almost logarithmically for years.[2]

Using recombinant methods, researchers have been able to locate the genetic DNA variations responsible for a number of devastating diseases. By the end of the 1980s, scientific leaders from around the world decided to go beyond these individual efforts to coordinate activities in a major initiative to map the human genome.[3] Having assigned responsibility for chromosomes to genetics centers, the architects of this activity in the national research directorates and in HUGO (the Human Genome Organization) expect to locate all 50-100,000 genes that make up the human genome within about five years, though it will take longer to ascertain the DNA sequences of the genes on the chromosomes. This work involves studying the genome not only of *homo sapiens* but also of other species, both to add to our understanding of genes generally and to aid in the development of methods to make human genome mapping easier and less expensive.

The origins of special concern about genetics

Given its connection not only with inheritance and family ties but also with what is "inherent" in each person, it is not surprising that genetics excites special concern among ethicists and policymakers. Furthermore, the very method of molecular genetics — which is to break the origins of human traits and characteristics down to tiny variations in DNA — consists of materialistic reductionism and propagates what for many people is the offensive notion that by possessing a list of DNA base-pairs one could "know" a person.

These aspects of molecular genetics help to explain the underlying anxiety that the subject produces, the sense that something especially worrisome is involved. But as far as human subjects research is concerned, I believe that the high level of attention devoted to the field owes much to more practical worries that emerged as the modern era of genetics was just dawning, in the early 1970s.

At that time, some researchers expressed concern that the techniques being used — specifically breaking apart DNA chains and splicing in DNA from another source — might have harmful effects on the environment and on human health. On the initiative of the scientists at a Gordon Research Conference in 1973,[4] a committee established by the United States National Academy of Sciences called in July 1974 for an international moratorium on certain categories of research.[5] Although the meeting held the following February at the Asilomar conference grounds near Monterey, California, lifted the cessation on most types of recombinant research and led the nations involved in this area of research to establish standards and procedures to minimize research risks, some critics of the moratorium have suggested that it permanently branded molecular genetics as "unusually hazardous" in the public's mind. Consequently, it is not surprising that genetics has received a great deal of attention from ethicists and policy-makers, at least some of it misguided.[6]

Beyond concern over physical risks, the application of molecular genetic techniques to human beings does raise profound issues but most of these are not, in my view, issues of human-subjects research. Rather, they relate to applications of genetic knowledge. For example, what will happen in the coming years as the range of genetic variations that can be diagnosed far exceeds the number for which any treatment is available?[7] This is a particularly worrisome issue regarding the identification of people who are apparently healthy but who have one or more genes that predispose them to "late-onset" diseases. Many "genetic diseases" are multifactorial, involving more than one gene as well as environmental factors. Therefore, early detection of the gene may in some cases permit prophylactic measures (change in diet, frequent medical monitoring for early symptoms, etc.), but in many instances early detection will merely mean untreatable worries.

Another issue raised by human applications of molecular genetics is the potential to "enhance" human capabilities, which could involve giving a person the genes responsible for the highest level of functioning (e.g., speed, agility, intelligence) found in other human beings, or giving from another species genes that would endow the human recipient with super-human abilities. (In addition to enhancement, genes from other species might be added for "debasement", that is the creation of a sub-human being with the ability to do repetitious or arduous tasks that humans were unwilling to undertake.) This issue poses basic questions about what is meant by "human nature" and by "disease", "normal", and "health". What seems to one observer to be a departure from normal functioning may be viewed as perfectly natural by another. Likewise, one person's "enhancement" can be another's "treatment of disease": if inserting growth-promoting genes to increase the height of a pituitary dwarf by 50 cm from 120 cm to 170 cm is "treatment", is adding a mere 40 cm to the height of a young, aspiring 170 cm-tall basketball player also "treatment" or is it "enhancement"?

Besides these questions of ends, molecular genetics also raises issues of means that fall within the ambit of guidelines for research with human subjects. Basic molecular research to map and sequence all human genes necessarily involves the use of human beings as the source of the DNA being examined; and then the application of information from genome mapping and other sources to the development of potential diagnostic, prophylactic, and therapeutic interventions, again depends on research with human beings. The question, then, is whether any aspects of these various forms of research are distinctive enough to deserve special attention when formulating ethical guidelines for research with human beings.

A basic issue raised by genetic research: defining "subjects"

Before turning to the draft revised CIOMS Guidelines, one needs a clearer understanding of the meaning of "human subject", the basic unit around which all the rest of the ethical analysis revolves. In ordinary experimentation, it is not difficult to tell who the subjects are: they are the people who are observed or manipulated for the purpose of producing generalizable knowledge.* Gray areas arise, of course, but the identity of the human subjects is usually assumed to be obvious; indeed, the draft CIOMS Guidelines appear not to define the term "subject".

Some questionable categories

Questions will sometimes arise about whether persons who are "normal controls" are subjects, especially if data about them are drawn from historical or clinical records. The usual response would be to regard them as subjects insofar as they might be affected by the research — such as through release of confidential information in a manner that identifies them. Especially in the case of randomized selection, it seems appropriate to regard those not on the experimental arm as subjects, even when they receive "standard therapy" in place of a placebo, because they have been deprived of whatever benefit may come from the intervention being tested. Even if that innovation is only available in the experiment and the controls would also not have gotten it had they not been in the experiment, they are still making a contribution by participating, and it can even be argued that they have been made "worse off", since participating in the research gave them an *ex ante* chance to obtain the benefit of the innovation being tested, from which they were excluded *ex post* by the randomization of subjects. This is one reason that randomized experiments often employ "cross over" designs, which give both groups a chance to receive the intervention being evaluated.

In addition to those directly manipulated, people who are affected indirectly are also subjects when such indirect effects are among the

---

* Regulations promulgated by the United States government define "human subject" as:
a living individual about whom an investigator... conducting [a systematic investigation designed to develop or contribute to generalizable knowledge] obtains (1) data through intervention or interaction with the individual, or (2) identifiable private information.
45 Code of Federal Regulations § 46.102(f).

matters being investigated — for example, when alterations are made in an environment in order to study the effects of these changes on living beings. However, not all people who are indirectly affected by an investigator's actions are subjects; for example, family members of a patient who receives innovative treatment may well be affected by both the process of the research and its outcome, yet they would not ordinarily be considered subjects unless their reactions are one of the topics under investigation.

Some complications added by genetic research

Genetic research markedly complicates the definition of "subject". First, consider genetic linkage studies that rely on polymorphisms. Such studies typically require the cooperation of a number of people across several generations in a family. Obviously, all those who are studied directly (those from whom biological samples are taken for genetic analysis) are subjects.

But the results of the study may also reveal information about family members who were unwilling to be studied. For example, if Grandpa agrees to have his blood taken for a test to reveal a genetic marker and it is found that his DNA does not have this marker (which is associated with a genetic disease in certain of his children and grandchildren), then it is likely that his wife (who was unwilling to have blood drawn) is the carrier of the disease. Does this make Grandma a subject of the research? (Of course, if the situation is reversed, the results indicate only that the father of the affected children probably carries the gene in question — that may be Grandpa or it may be someone else; likewise, if both Grandma and Grandpa are tested and neither carries the gene in question, the most likely explanation is usually that Grandpa is not the father of the children in question.)

The creation of information about the "obligate" status of genetic carriers is an example of the complications that genetic studies (molecular and traditional) can generate for guidelines for human-subjects research. Of course, giving meaning to the term *subject* is not an abstract task. Rather, words are defined for a purpose, and a change in the purpose may mean a change in what is encompassed by the definition. Thus, the question "Is Grandma a subject of research?" should be met with the reply, "Why do we want to know?".

If, for instance, the rule in question is that researchers may not reveal confidential information about subjects, it would seem appropriate to define people in Grandma's position as subjects: just as genetic information about those who have agreed to participate in the linkage study (e.g., Grandpa and his children and grandchildren) should not be revealed in a way that identifies them, so too Grandma's genetic status should be kept private (i.e., her name or other identifying characteristics should not be disclosed in any reports about the linkage study).

On the other hand, if the question is whether a person in Grandma's position is a subject within the meaning of a rule that requires consent from subjects before research can be conducted, one might well hold that such people are *not* subjects. Their unwillingness to participate means that their genetic material cannot be studied directly; they certainly have a right to refuse to this extent, to protect themselves against unconsented bodily invasions and unauthorized use of biological material derived from themselves. But this right does not extend to preventing researchers from studying other family members simply because doing so may produce data that (with varying degrees of certainty) reveal something about the non-subject's genetic status.

An even more complex example of the difficulties that molecular genetics can pose for the definition of *subject* arises from the prospect of germ-line gene therapy. Are the future offspring of a person who undergoes such an innovative intervention subjects of the research? In this case, any effect on them is contingent and not immediate, but if it does occur it is direct; moreover, such an effect is part of the very experiment and in all likelihood at least the children (and perhaps the grandchildren) would be studied by the researchers, probably both prenatally and postnatally. At the time of such studies either their parents or, once they are no longer children, they themselves would be asked for consent, and this aspect is comparable to any research. But such consent for particular tests on bodily fluids and the like pales beside the very fact that their genetic make-up will be altered by the intervention on their forebear. Is such a change in the genetic material that one inherits enough to make these hypothetical offspring "subjects" If so, the usual rule requiring their consent would mean that the research could not be done unless their forebear were considered an adequate and appropriate surrogate to give informed consent on their behalf.

Informed consent of subjects

Guideline 1: Individual informed consent

The requirement of informed consent is as important and as appropriate for genetics studies as for any research with human subjects. The question, as just suggested, is: who is a subject? I believe that there is little to be gained in terming the future hypothetical offspring a subject within the meaning of this principle. Permitting consent by a prospective subject or by a *"properly authorized representative"*, as the guideline does, focuses attention on individualized decision-making based on the particularized interests, values, etc., of the potential subject. Such a formulation makes sense when a parent (or other legally authorized representative) is deciding on a child's behalf. But it really makes no sense when an individual is deciding on behalf of a purely hypothetical entity, not merely in the next, but in some distant, generation.

The useless nature of the permission that might be sought from the potential subject of germ-line therapy on behalf of all his or her offspring is underlined by the fact that this person may at this time not only not have children but may be young and unmarried, with no clear thought of what it means to make decisions on behalf of a potential child. If the gene therapy proposed for the benefit of this person (perhaps the only means of genetic or other treatment that is possible) either risks an inadvertent effect on his or her gametes or is intended to have such an effect, can this person possibly consent on behalf of hypothetical future offspring? Is not this person's self-interest too great a conflict? An alternative scenario would be if potential parents were asked to consent to genetic manipulation of their gametes, or of a zygote created from their gametes, as a means of preventing a genetic disease in that child; would they also be the "properly authorized representatives" from whom it is appropriate to obtain consent on behalf of all their unborn — or even unconceived — child's offspring who would also carry the altered gene?

Rather than term future children, grandchildren, and so forth "subjects", it would seem more appropriate to treat this as a situation in which permission for the research ought to come from people in addition to the immediate subject. In the United States, for example, federally sponsored gene therapy must be approved by the Recombinant DNA Advisory Committee (RAC) and its Human Gene Therapy Subcommittee (HGTS), which advise the Director of the National Institutes of Health (NIH). Under the *Points to Consider for Human Gene Therapy*, these bodies "will not at present entertain proposals for germ line alterations".[8] This reflects a collective judgment that, at present, germ-line transmission of genetic changes would involve too great a risk to offspring.

The NIH review bodies thus serve the protective function for all future persons who might be affected by such a genetic alteration, since no one else exists who could play this role effectively. Furthermore, this protective role is undertaken not only to safeguard potential future individuals but also to protect society at large from the too rapid implementation of the biomedical capability, in effect, to interfere with the course of evolution. Unfortunately, the NIH committees have not gone beyond the conclusion that germ-line therapy would at this juncture be inappropriate for technical reasons (because of the risk that inserted genetic material might become harmful in offspring if it is not incorporated into the appropriate place on the chromosome). The ethical reasons for differentiating germ-line from somatic-cell therapy have been assumed to be obvious, when in fact they may prove to be difficult to spell out.

Were true "gene surgery" possible (that is, the precise replacement of a malfunctioning gene with the normal gene, in a manner that was stable during reproduction), it is not intuitively obvious why it is acceptable to cure a disease in an individual but not to avoid the occurrence of the disease in that individual's descendants. The greatest risk to society (and to the descendants) would be that the deleted allele had some unknown compensatory advantage or would have such an advantage under certain changes in the environment that would be more lethal to people who lacked this "abnormal" allele (in shorthand, the importance of hybrid vigor and genetic heterogeneity for a population). Depending on the condition and how lethal it is untreated, the potential harm from eliminating the gene in most or all patients *and their descendants* might well be outweighed by the benefit.

Other possible problems with germ-line interventions have not been well articulated. It is true that the development of germ-line techniques for use in narrow cases of the type just hypothesized would make it easier to make inherited characteristics that are not usually thought of as diseases; carried to the limit, this could amount to "designing" future generations. The problem with this argument is that it condemns all gene therapy, including somatic-cell therapy for otherwise untreatable lethal conditions: the knowledge developed in these treatments also provides building blocks for Orwellian forms of genetic alterations. Likewise, the ethical/religious objection that all forms of genetic modification tinker with nature in a way that only God is supposed to applies as much to somatic-cell as to germ-line therapy.

Guideline 2: Essential information for prospective research-subjects

The second guideline obliges investigators to present certain information to potential subjects before obtaining their consent; the implication is that, besides presenting such information, the investigator is also required to make good the promises implicit in this information. One point of particular importance in genetic studies is the obligation to make clear to subjects the duration of their involvement. When biological material is placed in a "gene bank", the subject becomes involved with genetic studies for an indefinite time, since future researchers may return to samples collected many years previously when new tests or knowledge would provide a basis for a new means or objective in reanalysing the samples. Thus, it is important that potential subjects understand and accept the potential for such reanalysis. If they are willing to have their cells checked for a particular genetic condition (perhaps because of its clinical relevance for members of their family) but unwilling to become the subject of future, as yet unspecified, studies, means should be readily available for the subjects to place restrictions on the use of any samples obtained, including keeping such samples from being placed in a bank.

The final point listed in the draft guideline as part of the information that must be communicated is that the subject is free to abstain or to withdraw from participation in the research at any time without penalty or loss of benefits to which he or she would otherwise be entitled.

Molecular genetic studies pose problems in fulfilling this "right to withdraw", under two scenarios. First are situations comparable to those that can arise with any therapy: once the innovative treatment has been applied, it may have permanent effects on the subject, who would thereafter be free "to withdraw from participation in the research" in the sense of no longer being studied or monitored but who might well *not* be free to withdraw in the sense of being returned to the *status quo ante*. In the case of gene therapy, the intention is to have permanent effects on at least a significant portion of the subject's cells. Unless the investigator is required to use only reversible methods and to have readily available means of reversal of whatever genetic changes are involved, the promise of subjects being able to withdraw can be seen as false or at best meaningless.

The second set of genetic experiments that pose difficulty are those in which a subject from whom biological material (leukocytes, fibroblasts) has been obtained decides to withdraw after the material has been placed in a data bank. As to the material still held by the bank, it might be difficult, but it would seem to be neither impossible nor even too onerous, to insist that such material be removed or at least made inaccessible for further research. But what of uses made of the material before the subject's decision to withdraw?

It would be onerous, indeed arbitrary, to insist that investigators be obliged to discard data already derived from (and perhaps already published) genetic analysis of a withdrawing subject's biological material. On the other hand, if the right to withdraw is to have any meaning, then the gene bank or other body that has biological samples that it distributes to laboratories for study ought to include with each sample a statement that, should the person from whom it was obtained withdraw consent, no further analysis may be performed on the material and the material itself would have to be either returned or destroyed. This restriction should be regarded as something that travels with the material, should the original laboratory pass on the material to others for study. Realistically, however, it is unlikely that such restrictions would be enforceable or universally obeyed in cases of second- or third-hand possession of a genetic sample. Since the sharing of the material may be very beneficial for science, an alternative, more stringent means of protecting the right to withdraw — namely, forbidding a researcher to pass along any material from a gene bank — should probably not be adopted as a universal requirement.

Guideline 3: Obligations of investigators regarding informed consent

Among an investigator's duties in obtaining informed consent, one is particularly sensitive in the context of genetic studies: that the investigator must make every effort to minimize the possibility of unjustified deception, undue influence and intimidation.

It is apparent that any deception that occurs is likely to emanate from an investigator's own behavior. (This is most often an issue in studies that are based on deceiving "naive" subjects about the investigators' true objectives in conducting the studies.) Hence it is reasonable to insist that investigators minimize deception. Undue influence and intimidation may also flow from what an investigator does or is — for example, when an investigator is also the physician to whom a subject feels beholden. But undue influence and intimidation sometimes arise from the actions of others, in which case an investigator may not be able "to minimize the possibility of ... undue influence and intimidation". Nonetheless, the investigator should not be able simply to ignore the outside sources of influence and intimidation, for to do so would be to obtain from a subject apparent consent that may have been involuntary and hence not consent at all.

This concern arises particularly in genetic linkage studies, which usually depend upon the cooperation of a sufficient number of family members from several generations. If the performance of a study is of particular concern to certain family members (such as those who are directly affected or those who face possible reproductive choices that would be affected by the outcome of the genetic analysis), investigators must be alert to the danger that these family members will put pressure on others to participate. The strategy for avoiding pressure of this type is more complex than the usual self-denying requirement that the investigator assure subjects that their decision whether to participate will not affect their therapeutic relationship. In the case of a genetic linkage study, the investigator ought routinely to explore with potential subjects their motivation for participation. Obviously the desire to help a relative is not an automatic disqualification; rather than showing involuntariness, such a motive may reflect a high level of altruism and empathy. Thus, rather than a special rule, what is needed is simply a reminder of the need to probe for motivation and to find ways to protect subjects who are actually reluctant or unwilling to participate in the study but who have been unduly pressured by others to consent.

Guideline 5: Research involving children

Although it is not elaborated in the commentary section, the first requirement of this draft guideline is that investigators must ensure that there is no valid alternative to the use of children. This issue will arise frequently with gene therapy, because many of the diseases for which such therapy is likely to be attempted are lethal early in life. For these diseases the requirement of "no valid alternative" will be met. Even in these cases, however, the notion of a valid alternative would seem to encompass a requirement that the disease in question not be susceptible to an effective and not too burdensome existing treatment. When such treatment does exist, it would seem reasonable to delay testing of gene therapy for the disease until the basic techniques of gene therapy are well understood and generally accepted. For example, phenylketonuria would probably be an inappropriate disease for an early trial of gene therapy, since effective dietary therapy is already available.

When both minors and adults suffer from a disease, at what point is it appropriate to permit minors to be subjects? Although it is understandable to regard anything labeled gene *therapy* as potentially beneficial and therefore to be concerned lest children be discriminated against in being kept out of the experiment, there are good reasons for adhering to the basic rule and turning first to subjects who are able to consent on their own behalf.

Guideline 11: Pregnant and nursing women as research subjects

The major example of the use of genetic data prophylactically has been in reproduction, both in genetic counseling of potentially at-risk couples who are deciding whether to have children and in prenatal diagnosis. The former does not raise any unique problems, though the sometimes complex and probabilistic information that must be conveyed in the counseling process can add to the difficulty of obtaining truly informed consent. On the other hand, the tradition of "noncoercive and nondirective counseling" in this field,[9] means that counselors profess greater allegiance to the norm of patient autonomy in this field than they have done in other areas of medical practice.

The second "preventive" use of genetics in reproduction has been through prenatal diagnosis. Depending on one's viewpoint, this subject can be addressed under either Guideline 11, if one focuses on the pregnant woman as the subject, or Guideline 5, if one focuses on the fetus as a child-subject-to-be. Furthermore, the draft guidelines suggest that separate attention may be given to research with embryos and fetuses, in which case prenatal genetic diagnosis might also be encompassed by guidelines developed under that heading.

However the guidelines are formulated, the special issue raised here is whether a pregnant woman — alone or with her mate — will have full freedom to participate in research aimed at applying genetic knowledge to determine the health status of her fetus. Some critics of prenatal diagnosis have characterized it as a "search and destroy" mission, in which the interests of the pregnant woman are adverse to those of the fetus. This characterization carried greater resonance in the early years of the procedure, in the 1970s, when prenatal diagnosis usually involved amniocentesis late in the fourth month of gestation, followed by three to four weeks' wait while cytogenetic studies were carried out on the cultured fetal cells; this meant that a fetus was often nearing the end of the second trimester by the time information was available on which to make a decision about continuing the pregnancy. Today other methods of gathering fetal cells — including from maternal serum — permit many diseases to be diagnosed quite early in pregnancy.

Furthermore, in nearly all cases (roughly 95%), prenatal diagnosis is not followed by abortion; indeed, the reassuring information that a prenatal test can provide may prevent an abortion that a woman would otherwise have rather than take even a small risk of bearing a child with a severe abnormality, especially when she is aware of the risk because of previously having given birth to an affected child.

The upshot is that Guideline 11 is probably adequate to address the considerations. Provided that adequate preclinical research has occurred and that diagnostic tests have been carried as far as they can on non-pregnant women, eventually there will be no valid alternative to the use of pregnant women in the development of genetic methods of prenatal diagnosis.

Confidentiality of data

Guideline 12: Safeguarding confidentiality

The basic requirement of confidentiality of data is fully applicable to genetic studies. Indeed, the inherent nature of genetic information (as distinct from information about acquired characteristics or diseases) and people's present feeling of high sensitivity about the information underline just how important this guideline will be for research on genetic conditions.

One particular concern regarding genetic data — which may also arise *vis-à-vis* data about nongenetic diseases — is the effect on individuals when they possess data about themselves that they may be, or may believe themselves to be, obliged to disclose to others whom either disclosure or nondisclosure would harm. Suppose that genetic tests will reveal a person's susceptibility to a fatal illness in middle life. Without knowing about the susceptibility, a person would have nothing to disclose about it when seeking life insurance. But a subject who participates in a study that turns up evidence of susceptibility must then either disclose this suceptibility when asked (and risk being denied insurance) or withhold it (and risk having an insurance claim disallowed later on grounds of fraud).

When such disclosures occur, they do not result directly from the act of the investigator and so might seem to fall outside this guideline. To be consistent with the spirit of the guideline, however, the "precautions" that an investigator should take to protect potential subjects ought to include at a minimum warning them if any of the information that the study is likely to produce would affect their insurability.

Conclusion

Ethicists will continue to identify and analyse many difficult or perhaps intractable problems raised by molecular genetics. Some of those problems — principally, whether, and if so how, gene therapy that will produce inheritable changes should be conducted — are tied up in the standards and procedures established to govern research involving human subjects. But, for the most part, the difficulties posed by developments in human genetics are conceptual and relate to clinical and other uses of the techniques, not to the methods by which they are established through research involving human subjects. Thus, it is my belief that the guidelines do not need to treat genetic research separately, though some of the points raised in this paper could usefully be added to the commentary sections of the guidelines.

References

1. See generally Bernard D. Davis, ed., *The genetic revolution: scientific prospects and public perceptions* (1991), especially Theodore Friedmann, Molecular Medicine, at pp. 132-151.
2. Victor A. McKusick, *Mendelian inheritance in man* (1988).
3. See, e.g., Office of Technology Assessment, *Mapping our genes: genome projects — how big? how fast?* (1988).
4. See Maxine Singer & Dieter Soll, Guidelines for DNA Hybrid Molecules, *Science* 181 (1973): 1114.
5. National Academy of Sciences — National Research Council, Committee on Recombinant DNA Molecules. Potential Biohazards of Recombinant DNA Molecules, *Science* 185 (1974): 303.
6. See A.M. Capron, Which Ills to Bear?: Reevaluating the "Threat" of Modern Genetics, *Emory Law Journal* 39 (Summer 1990): 665-696.
7. See, e.g., Nancy Wexler, The Oracle of DNA, in: *Social Policy and Molecular Genetics* (1990) 429-442.
8. Points to Consider for Proposals for the Transfer of Recombinant DNA into the Genome of Human Subjects, "Introduction, Point (7)", 55 *Federal Register* 7444 (1st March 1990).
9. See, E.g. Aubrey Milunsky, Genetic Counseling: Principles and Practices in A. Milunsky, ed., *The Prevention of Genetic Disease and Mental Retardation* (1975), pp. 64-71.

THE REGULATION OF RESEARCH ON HUMAN SUBJECTS: A DECADE OF PROGRESS

Richard J. Kelly, Sev S. Fluss, and Frank Gutteridge*

> *"... respect for human rights in human experimentation demands that we see persons as unique, as ends in themselves."*
>
> — Elie Wiesel, Nobel
> Peace Prize Laureate

Introduction

For many years the Council for International Organizations of Medical Sciences (CIOMS) has promoted international debate on the public-policy, ethical, moral, and legal implications of advances in medicine and biomedical sciences. As early as 1976, in cooperation with WHO, CIOMS initiated in-depth work on the ethical conduct of biomedical research involving human subjects. In particular, it consulted national health administrations, faculties of medicine, and experts representing a wide variety of backgrounds in developed and developing countries alike. Particular focus was placed on a Joint WHO/CIOMS Project for the Development of Guidelines for Ethical Review Procedures for Research Involving Human Subjects. Perhaps the culminating event in the process that led to the development of Guidelines on this subject was the XVth CIOMS Round Table, on Human Experimentation and Medical Ethics, held in Manila on 13-16 September 1981. At that Conference, and at the request of CIOMS, one of us (SSF) presented a paper[1] which sought to review all available international documents and national legislation, as well as codes and other measures, that addressed the key elements of the proposed guidelines. The paper demonstrated that, at the time, relatively few Member States of WHO had enacted legislation or had taken other measures to protect the human subjects of medical experimentation. Since September 1981, a significant number of countries (including several developing countries) have adopted legislation or taken other measures to regulate experimentation on human subjects. It is clear that various countries have been influenced by international developments, including, in particular, the successive versions of the World Medical Association's Declaration of Helsinki and the 1982

---

* Mr. R.J. Kelly is a medical/law student at Stanford University, Palo Alto, California; at the time of preparation of this paper he was an intern with the Health Legislation unit, WHO. Mr. S.S. Fluss is Chief, Health Legislation unit, WHO. Mr. F. Gutteridge was formerly Director, Legal Division, WHO, and is currently a consultant to CIOMS. Any views expressed are those of the authors and not necessarily those of WHO, except where clearly indicated.

WHO/CIOMS Proposed International Guidelines for Biomedical Research Involving Human Subjects.

There has also been increased international attention, not least within certain United Nations bodies, to the ethical conduct of human experimentation, and the matter has received attention in certain of the bioethics "summits" organized by the seven major market-economy industrialized countries (the so-called "G-7").

The decade since the publication of the 1982 Proposed International Guidelines has moreover witnessed significant advances in the medical and biomedical sciences, which have modified our understanding of ethical conduct in the more traditional settings, while opening up entirely new vistas and new ethical issues. The HIV/AIDS pandemic, a greater sensitivity to the need to offer particular protection for vulnerable social groups, and other factors have influenced our ethical stance on whether pregnant women, children, prisoners, etc. should be subjects of human experimentation. New therapeutic modalities, such as somatic gene therapy, and pioneering work with fetal tissues and embryos, have raised new ethical issues that scarcely existed a decade ago.[2]

This paper seeks to update the information presented at the Manila Conference in September 1981, and also to examine how international texts and national legislation have already dealt with some of the key elements covered in the first draft of the 1992 International Ethical Guidelines for Biomedical Research Involving Human Subjects. Like its predecessor, this paper cannot aspire to be as comprehensive as it no doubt could and should be. The authors are constrained by the fact that WHO's Health Legislation unit has regular access to the legislation of only about one-half of the Organization's 179 Member States (valuable additional materials have been made available by WHO's Global Programme on AIDS and by CIOMS). Furthermore, among those Member States that do report legislative information to the Organization under Article 63 of WHO's Constitution, some of the legislation, guidelines, codes, and other measures are so voluminous that space constraints have necessitated a choice to be made by the authors. Wherever possible, reference is further made to all available legislative and other instruments and the equivalent.

International Developments

There are now a significant number of international instruments and documents that establish guidance for the regulation of experimentation on human subjects. Chronologically, the first modern international document, the Nuremberg Code of 1947, was drawn up shortly after the Second World War in response to the wholly unethical medical experiments performed on unconsenting prisoners, purportedly in the interests of "military medical science". The judges in what is generally termed the Nuremberg Doctors' Trial, in their condemnation of these experiments and of the guilty defendants, set out 10 conditions for the ethical conduct of experimentation on human subjects. The document was aimed at protecting the integrity of the experimental subject and endorsed human experimentation, provided the criteria set forth in the Code were complied with. The Nuremberg Code has been criticized by certain specialists on two grounds, however. First, the Code does not distinguish between different types of biomedical experimentation and, second, the Code makes the subject's legal capacity to consent a prerequisite to experimentation, thus excluding from participating in research many people who might benefit from the results obtained, including children, the mentally ill, and others who are unable to give legal consent.[3]

The World Medical Association

The Declaration of Helsinki, originally adopted in 1964 by the World Medical Association, has been of considerable importance in the formulation of national legislation and codes of conduct. The Declaration, revised in Tokyo in 1975 ("Helsinki II"), in Venice in 1983 ("Helsinki III"), and again in Hong Kong in 1989 ("Helsinki IV"), is a comprehensive international statement on the ethics of human experimentation. It established a distinction between therapeutic and non-therapeutic experimentation (one of the early national texts to establish such a distinction was the United Kingdom Medical Research Council's Statement: "Responsibility in Investigations on Human Subjects" (1962-63; a revised version is expected to appear before the end of 1992); it is noteworthy that one of the earliest United States texts dealing with research on human subjects, the Memorandum of 26 February 1953 of the Department of Defense, addressed non-therapeutic experimentation only). Moreover, the Declaration, unlike the Nuremberg Code, allows experimentation on legally incompetent persons.

The Council for International Organizations of Medical Sciences

The 1982 WHO/CIOMS Proposed International Guidelines for Biomedical Research Involving Human Subjects were a logical, progressive development of the Declaration of Helsinki. As the preamble clearly states, the Guidelines are not merely a repetition of the principles set out in the Declaration of Helsinki, but were promulgated to make concrete suggestions for applying the principles of the Declaration, especially in developing countries.

- Since the publication of the 1982 Proposed International Guidelines, CIOMS in cooperation with WHO has continued to prepare important documents relating to human experimentation. Thus, in 1991, CIOMS published *International Guidelines for Ethical Review of Epidemiological Studies*.[4] These Guidelines are intended to assist investigators and institutions as well as regional and national authorities in the development of standards for the ethical review of epidemiological studies. It is the first international document to provide a foundation for the ethical regulation of epidemiological research and investigations. The section on assessment of safety and quality is reproduced below:

41. All drugs and devices under investigation must meet adequate standards of safety. In this respect, many countries lack resources to undertake independent assessment of technical data. A governmental multidisciplinary committee with authority to co-opt experts is the most suitable body for assessing the safety and quality of medicines, devices and procedures. Such a committee should include clinicians, pharmacologists, statisticians and epidemiologists, among others; for epidemiological studies, epidemiologists occupy a position of obvious significance. Ethical review procedures should provide for consultation with such a committee.

The World Psychiatric Association

The Declaration of Hawaii II (1992) of the World Psychiatric Association includes ethical rules for research involving psychiatric patients. Article 9 points out that participation of patients is required to increase and propagate psychiatric knowledge and skill, and refers to informed consent, voluntary participation, full information, the relationship between risks and benefits, and freedom to withdraw from any research programme. Article 10 requires the psychiatrist to stop all research programs that may evolve contrary to the principles of the Declaration.

The United Nations

The United Nations has also been active in developing instruments that, *inter alia*, seek to regulate certain types of human experimentation. Thus, on 2 April 1991, the United Nations General Assembly (by resolution 45/113) endorsed a set of "United Nations Rules for the Protection of Juveniles Deprived of their Liberty". These Rules include the following paragraph:

53. Medicines should be administered only for necessary treatment on medical grounds and, when possible, after having obtained the informed consent of the juvenile concerned... Juveniles shall never be testees in the experimental use of drugs and treatment...

- On 17 December 1991, the United Nations General Assembly (by resolution 46/119) endorsed a set of "Principles for the Protection of Persons with Mental Illness and for the Improvement of Mental

Health Care". Principle 11 is entitled "Consent to treatment" and includes the following paragraph:

15. Clinical trials and experimental treatment shall never be carried out on any patient without informed consent, except that a patient who is unable to give informed consent may be admitted to a clinical trial or given experimental treatment, but only with the approval of a competent, independent review body specifically constituted for this purpose.

The G-7 countries

On 6-10 April 1987, the G-7 countries convened their Fourth International Summit Conference on Bioethics, in Ottawa, on the theme "Ethics Standards for Research Across Nations and Cultures". The Conference participants consisted of 26 leading experts who had been selected by the Heads of State or Heads of Government of the seven countries, by the European Community, and by CIOMS. They formulated a number of recommendations aimed at establishing international standards for research on human subjects. In particular, they recommended that a broad range of disciplines be represented on ethical review committees. They also endorsed, under narrowly prescribed conditions, research involving children, but did not achieve consensus on research with human embryos. Their recommendations included compensation for research-related injury, special considerations for novel therapies, standards for industrial research, and ethical selection of research topics.

At the invitation of the organizers, WHO prepared an information document for the Conference entitled "Human experimentation: a concise overview of international instruments and legislation, guidelines, ethical codes, etc. in the seven Summit countries".

The Council of Europe

In February 1990 the Committee of Ministers of the Council of Europe adopted Recommendation No. R (90) 3 to member states concerning medical research on human beings. This Recommendation established a set of 16 principles addressing such aspects as: informed consent; experiments involving children, the mentally ill, pregnant and nursing women, and prisoners; emergency situations where the patient is unable to give prior informed consent; confidentiality; safety of the research; ethical review procedures; etc. The following extracts specifically address the compensation issue:

Principle 13

1. Potential subjects of medical research should not be offered any inducement which compromises free consent. Persons undergoing

131

medical research should not gain any financial benefit. However, expenses and any financial loss may be refunded and in appropriate cases a modest allowance may be given for any inconvenience inherent in the medical research.

2. If the person undergoing research is legally incapacitated, his legal representatives should not receive any form of remuneration whatever, except for the refund of their expenses.

Principle 14

1. Persons undergoing medical research and/or their dependants should be compensated for injury and loss caused by the medical research.

2. Where there is no existing system providing compensation for the persons concerned, states should ensure that sufficient guarantees for such compensation are provided.

3. Terms and conditions which exclude or limit, in advance, compensation to the victim should be considered to be null and void.

The Explanatory Memorandum to the Recommendation has not yet been published, but it is available in the form of a document. The following is an extract from the Introduction:

1. The need to ensure that there is a proper balance in the rules on medical research on human beings between the respect of a person and the benefit of the progress of the medical sciences requires the weighing up of interests which are often contradictory and difficult to take into account owing to the continuous scientific and technical progress.

The path to be followed in this field is based on Human Rights as understood by member States of the Council of Europe and is reflected, in particular, in the Convention for the protection of human rights and fundamental freedoms, even though medical research is not expressly mentioned.

The ethical, legal and clinical debates on experimentation are no longer confined to specialised groups but now include the general public.

In addition, research based on pharmaceutical products is not the only field which gives rise to problems. Account should also be taken of problems created by the adoption of new methods of treatment, diagnosis, prevention, etc. which require research on human beings.

An earlier development under the auspices of the Council of Europe was the publication, in April 1983, of a report entitled "Problems Related to the Conduct and Control of Clinical Trials". It should also be mentioned that, in September 1986, the Parliamentary Assembly of the Council of Europe adopted Recommendation 1046 (1986) on reproductive technologies. In this Recommendation, Governments of Member States of the Council of Europe are recommended to prohibit, *inter alia*, research on viable human embryos and experimentation on living human embryos, whether viable or not. On 2 February 1989, the same body adopted Recommendation 1100 (1989) "on the use of human embryos and foetuses in scientific research". Owing to space constraints, the preambular and operative paragraphs of this Recommendation cannot be reproduced here. There is an Appendix entitled "Scientific research and/or experimentation on human gametes, embryos and foetuses and donation of such human material", in which the subject is discussed under the following rubrics: A. On gametes; B. On live pre-implantation embryos; C. On dead pre-implantation embryos; D. On post-implantation embryos or live foetuses *in utero*; E. On post-implantation embryos or live foetuses outside the uterus; F. On dead embryos or foetuses; G. Applications of scientific research to the human being in the fields of health and heredity; and H. Donation of human embryological material.

• In 1989 the Council of Europe published an Information Document entitled *Human Artificial Procreation*. This contains a series of Principles developed by the Council of Europe's ad hoc Committee of Experts on Bioethics (CAHBI). The following is the text of Principle 16, and an extract from Principle 17 under rubric VII, "Acts and procedures carried out on embryos":

Principle 16

The fertilisation of ova in vitro and the obtaining of embryos by lavage shall not be permitted for research purposes.

Principle 17

1.   No act or procedure shall be permitted on any embryo in vitro *other than those intended for the benefit of the embryo and for observational studies which do no harm to the embryo.*

2. When a state allows, in addition, investigative and experimental procedures other than those mentioned in the preceding paragraph for a preventive, diagnostic or therapeutic purpose for grave diseases of embryos, it shall require that the following conditions be fulfilled:

a. the purpose cannot be achieved by any other method; and

b. the embryo shall not be used after fourteen days from fertilisation, any period of storage by freezing or by any other means not included; and c. the consent of the couple has been given according to paragraph 3 of Principle 8 and, if the embryo has resulted from fertilisation in vitro *using donors' gametes, their consent shall also be required; and*

d. a properly consituted multidisciplinary ethical committee has given its approval."

- On 22-24 January 1992 the ad hoc Committee of Experts on Biothics convened the first meeting of its Working Party on Medical Research (CAHBI-CO-GT2); its terms of reference are to develop a "draft Protocol on medical research on human beings" (this will be one of the protocols to the proposed Framework Convention on Bioethics, now being developed under the auspices of the Council of Europe). It would be premature to deal with this development in any detail at this stage.

The European Communities

In May 1987 the Commission of the European Communities issued a "Note for Guidance" entitled "Recommended Basis for the Conduct of Clinical Trials of Medicinal Products in the European Community". In paragraph 8.2 of this text, it is stated that the ethical evaluation of research protocols should be undertaken in accordance with the provisions of Helsinki III. In September 1988 two parallel documents were issued, entitled "Clinical Investigation of Medicinal Products in Children" and "Clinical Investigation of Medicinal Products in the Elderly". Both of these texts address ethical issues.

- In 1988 a "Note for Guidance" entitled "Good Clinical Practice for Trials on Medicinal Products in the European Community" was issued under the auspices of the Committee for Proprietary Medicinal Products Working Party on Efficacy of Medicinal Products. Chapter 1 of this Note is entitled "Protection of trial subjects and consultation of ethics committees". Paragraph 1.8 of this Chapter reads as follows:

The principles of informed consent in the current revision [sic] of the Helsinki Declaration should be implemented in each clinical trial.

- The endorsement of the Declaration of Helsinki recurs in certain Council directives. Thus, Council Directive 91/507/EEC of 19 July 1991, which amended the Annex to Council Directive 75/318/EEC of 20 May 1975, contains a substantial amount of information concerning the clinical documentation that is required to accompany applications for marketing authorizations (under Council Directive 65/65/EEC of 26 January 1965). The following is an extract:

1.2 All clinical trials shall be carried out in accordance with the ethical principles laid down in the current revision of the Declaration of Helsinki. In principle, the freely given informed consent of each trial subject shall be obtained and documented.

- On 23 January 1991 the Directorate-General for the Internal Market and Industrial Affairs issued a document entitled "Discussion paper on the need for a directive on clinical trials". No information is available on the current status of the debate on this discussion paper.

- Reference should also be made to the resolution adopted on 16 March 1989 by the European Parliament on the ethical and legal problems of genetic engineering. This resolution addresses research on embryos and various other matters that are relevant to the research context, including military research and application.

The Nordic Committee on Medicines

This Committee functions under the auspices of the Nordic Council, an organization of which the Member States are Denmark, Finland, Iceland, Norway, and Sweden. The Committee has published a guide to human experimentation in the context of clinical drug trials. In December 1989, it issued *Good Clinical Trial Practice*, which contains, *inter alia*, provisions dealing with informed consent, prior review of experimental protocols by ethics committees, and insurance of experimental subjects against accidental injury.

The Northern Nurses' Federation

The 1990 Report of the Central Scientific-Ethical Committee of Denmark includes the text of the English version of the Northern Nurses' Federation's Ethical Guidelines for Nursing Research in the Nordic Countries. It is noteworthy that the definition of research contained in the Guidelines is that formulated by the Organisation for Economic Co-operation and Development, viz.: "scientific research is considered as research if its primary aim is to create new knowledge, develop new products and processes or improve existing products and processes."

The Conférence Internationale des Ordres et des Organismes d'Attributions Similaires

This body, whose membership comprises the General Medical Council (United Kingdom), the French *Conseil National de l'Ordre des Médecins*, and equivalent bodies in the other Member States of the European Community, adopted Principles of European Medical Ethics in January 1987. Articles 18-21 of the Principles acknowledge that human experimentation is necessary for progress in medicine but require all experimental protocols involving human subjects to be transmitted to an ethical review committee prior to execution. In addition, the investigator must obtain each subject's informed consent. The official English translation of these Articles reads as follows:

> *Article 18. Progress in the field of medicine is based on research which may not be undertaken without experimentation which has a direct bearing on humans.*
>
> *Article 19. Details of all proposed experimentation involving patients must first be submitted to an ethical committee which is independent of the research team for opinions and advice.*
>
> *Article 20. The free and informed consent of any person who is to be involved in a research project must be obtained after he has first been sufficiently informed of the aims, methods and expected benefits as well as the risks and potential problems, and of his right not to take part in experiments (or other research) and to withdraw from participation at any time.*
>
> *Article 21. The doctor may not link biomedical research with medical treatment, with a view to developing medical knowledge, except insofar as that biomedical research is justified by a potential diagnostic or therapeutic aid which will be relevant to his patient.*

European Medical Research Councils

In June 1988 this body published a set of "guidelines for the conduct of research on gene therapy in man and member countries". The Medical Research Councils represented were those of Austria, Denmark, the Federal Republic of Germany, Finland, France, the Netherlands, Norway, Spain, Sweden, Switzerland, and the United Kingdom. The following is the Summary:

> *1. The purpose of gene therapy currently under consideration is the correction of genetic defects; attempts to enhance general human characteristics should not be contemplated. Only somatic cell gene therapy, resulting in non-heritable changes to particular body tissues, should be contemplated. Germline therapy, for introduction of heritable genetic modifications, is not acceptable. Further technical improvements in the expression of transferred genes in somatic cells will be necessary before successful gene therapy can be achieved even in animal models; in the meantime trials in man are not justified.*
>
> *2. The most appropriate "candidate" genetic diseases for early investigation of treatment by gene therapy are single-gene disorders for which the affected gene and its regulation have been characterized.*

3. In the near future, it is likely that success in the introduction of normal genes into human cells will be achieved through the use of disabled retrovirus vectors, although other techniques may advance rapidly. Much further work is required in the development of safe species-specific and tissue-specific retrovirus vectors. The methods of gene introduction should not result in the spread of gene or vector to other tissues within the body or to people in contact with the patient. The possibility of a significant increase in the predisposition of the patient to cancer should be evaluated in considering the risks and benefits of the treatment. In addition, the expression and regulation of the gene inserted should be stable and sufficient to ensure a therapeutic effect.

4. General ethical considerations applicable to any new clinical treatment apply to human gene therapy and, in the first instance, will require assessment in individual cases. In the near future it is likely that such therapy will be clinically justified in particular patients with invariably fatal or life-threatening diseases, provided informed consent is obtained and no alternative treatment is available.

5. A national body should consider all proposals for human gene therapy and ensure the application of agreed national guidelines. Early trials should be monitored by a central body.

National Developments

The African Region

Algeria. On 31 July 1990, Law No. 85-05 of 16 February 1985 on health protection and promotion was amended by Law No. 90-17; some of the new provisions dealt with ethical review of human experimentation. Thus, a National Commission on the Ethics of the Health Sciences was established, its terms of reference including providing guidance and issuing opinions and recommendations on human experimentation.

Burundi. The Ministry of Public Health has established an AIDS/ Sexually Transmitted Diseases Research Committee, responsible for considering the ethical appropriateness of research proposals involving human subjects. WHO has been informed that this Committee requires that, prior to experimentation on human subjects, investigators must obtain from animal models data that demonstrate the safety and efficacy of the product being tested. In the case of externally sponsored research, the Committee requires that the proposed experimentation has received approval for testing on human subjects from the national regulatory authorities in the sponsoring country.

Côte d'Ivoire. The Minister of Public Health and Population has established a Research Committee, responsible for reviewing and approving all research protocols involving human subjects. The Committee addresses all ethical issues on a case-by-case basis, although there appear to be no special requirements for obtaining informed consent from the human subjects participating in the research project.

Malawi. There are at present three ethical review committees involved in the clearance of HIV/AIDS research: the Health Sciences Research Committee; the National Research Committee; and the National AIDS Committee. A special committee (the Medicines Committee of the Pharmacy, Medicines and Poisons Board) deals with the registration of compounds and with clinical investigations, and liaises with the three other committees. There appear to be procedures for obtaining informed consent.

South Africa. The 1987 Revised Edition of the South African Medical Research Council's *Ethical Considerations in Medical Research* contains a number of sections that deal with aspects of human experimentation. Discussion in this revised edition is devoted to issues of informed consent and experimentation involving embryos, fetuses, pregnant women, minors, the institutionalized mentally infirm, and prisoners as well as sections relating to research on recombinant DNA and gene therapy.

- Reference should also be made to the South African Committee for Genetic Experimentation (SAGENE), established in December 1978 and most recently reconstituted by a Government Notice of 15 May 1992. Its terms of reference include advising "any person and/or body concerned with research into or the application of recombinant DNA...".

Uganda. Although no legislation exists, the Government of Uganda, probably acting through the Minister of Health and the Director of Medical Services, is reported to ensure that research involving human subjects conforms to the ethical standards of the Declaration of Helsinki.

United Republic of Tanzania. There is no official national ethics committee responsible for medical research, and there is no legislation that deals with human experimentation. It has been reported that an *ad hoc* research expert committee advises the Chief Medical Officer, who then takes the final decision on the approval of research protocols.

Zaire. Research protocols using human volunteers are generally approved by local ethical committees. It appears, however, that these local committees do not necessarily have Government endorsement.

Zambia. All proposed research projects and trials involving human subjects are subject to the authorization of the Research and Ethics Committee set up within the Ministry of health.

Zimbabwe. There are detailed provisions concerning the conduct of clinical trials in the Drugs and Allied Substances Control Amendment Act, 1987. No such trials may be conducted without the written authorization of the Drugs Control Council. Sec. 15E of the new Part IA introduced into the principal Act by the new statute lays down that where the Council is granted written authorization for the conduct of a clinical trial of a drug, no such trial may take place until, among other requirements: in the case of a drug for the treatment of adult persons, the voluntary written consents of all such persons taking part in the clinical trial have been freely obtained; and in the case of a drug for the treatment of minors or persons under legal disability, the voluntary written consents of their parents or legal guardians, as the case may be, have been freely obtained.

The South-East Asia Region

India. The authors are unaware of any developments in India during the decade under review. It appears that the *Ethical Considerations Involved in Research on Human Subjects*, issued in February 1980 by the Indian Council of Medical Research, remain valid.

Nepal. The Nepal Medical Research Council Act, 2047 (1991) provided for the establishment and management of this Council. Under Sec. 11 of this Act, any person or institution intending to conduct research on health-related matters is under the obligation to obtain the Council's permission. In giving such permission, the Council is empowered to impose such conditions as may be prescribed.

Sri Lanka. WHO has been informed that National Guidelines for the Conduct of Human Biomedical Research are in preparation. As early as 1981 an ethical review committee was established at the Faculty of Medicine of the University of Colombo; as of 1992, all of the faculties of medicine in the country have such committees, as has the Bandaranaike Memorial Ayurvedic Research Institute. It appears that decisions by these committees are based on the 1982 WHO/ CIOMS Proposed International Guidelines, as well as on Helsinki I and Helsinki II. In June 1991 the National Resources, Energy, and Science Authority (NARESA) established a Technical Advisory Committee on Ethical Conduct in Research. It is understood that its functions are: (*a*) to assist NARESA in regard to ethical matters pertaining to scientific research; and (*b*) to draft national guidelines for the conduct of scientific research, including medical research.

Thailand. There is no legislation on human experimentation in Thailand. The Ministry of Health did at one stage propose draft legislation on human experimentation, designed to establish a mechanism at both national and institutional levels to define studies involving human subjects and to ensure that they would be carried out with all due concern and respect for the safety of research subjects. However, the next Government did not pursue the matter and no attempt has yet been made to reintroduce the legislation. The Ministry of Public Health has established a Subcommittee on Ethical Review of Research Studies to look into the issue. Furthermore, the Board of the Medical Council has issued a Code of Ethics, in effect since 9 June 1983. The provisions dealing with human reproduction are as follows:

1. A medical practitioner who performs human experimentation must have the consent of the subjects and must be available to protect them from any risk that may arise in the course of such experimentation.

2. A medical practitioner must deal with the human subjects in the same manner as he deals with his or her patients in medical practice as provided in Chapter III [Medical practice] of this Code, mutatis mutandis.

3. A medical practitioner shall be responsible for any risk or injury to human subjects due to the progress of the experiment, and without any fault on the part of the subjects themselves.[a]

The Region of the Americas[b]

Bolivia. The Code of Medical Ethics of the Association of Physicians of Bolivia, dated 11 May 1986, includes some general provisions on experimentation.

Brazil. By an Order dated 13 April 1982, a Special Commission to Study and Propose Regulations on Biomedical Research Involving Human Subjects was established. Its terms of reference were to examine and propose: (*a*) the basic regulations to be applicable to biomedical research involving human subjects; (*b*) the procedures to be adopted to ensure compliance with the proposed Regulations; and (*c*) the translation into Portuguese, with a view to official adoption, of Helsinki II and the WHO/CIOMS Proposed International Guidelines for Biomedical Research Involving Human Subjects.

---

[a] The authors acknowledge the kind assistance of Dr V. Eungprabhanth, Director of the Program Promoting the Medical, Environmental, Health and Scientific Law Research Centre, Mahidol University, Bangkok, in the preparation of this information.

[b] In the preparation of this section of the paper the authors were greatly aided by a paper published by D.S. LaVertu and A.M. Linares in the *Bulletin of the Pan American Health Organization* 1990; 24(4): 469-79.

Canada. In 1978 the Medical Research Council of Canada (MRC) established a Standing Committee on Ethics in Experimentation; this Committee reviewed and prepared an update of the 1978 MRC Guidelines for the Protection of Human Subjects in Research. In November 1987 the MRC published its Guidelines on Research Involving Human Subjects. All research funded by the MRC is required to comply with these Guidelines, which contain eight chapters covering, inter alia, the following topics: the nature of human research; evaluation of risks and benefits; special types of research, including genetic engineering, pilot studies, clinical trials, and transplantation; and principles of informed consent, with sections dealing with inducements, continuing consent, deception, cross-cultural studies, children, incompetent adults, and research with embryos and fetuses. Also addressed are issues of confidentiality and the implementation of ethical responsibilities, including the composition of ethical review boards, and the submission of proposed research protocols for review by these boards.

- In May 1992, a Report on Research Involving Children was issued. It was prepared by the Consent Panel Task Force of the National Council on Bioethics in Human Research (with the support of the Canadian Paediatric Society). It is understood that the Report concludes that "research involving children [is] not only permissible, but obligatory, under certain conditions".

- In April 1983 the Canadian Nurses Association issued Ethical Guidelines for Nursing Research Involving Human Subjects. These Guidelines, stated to be based on the Canadian Nurses Association Code of Ethics, are classed under the following rubrics: I. The scientific merit of the research; II. Human subject consent, protection and confidentiality; and III. The setting where research is done.

- In December 1985 the Health Protection Branch of the Department of National Health and Welfare issued Guidelines for the Conduct of Clinical Investigations, intended for use by drug manufacturers in connection with the implementation of the relevant provisions of the Food and Drugs Act and the Food and Drugs Regulations. The Guidelines cover such aspects as: the responsibility of the investigator; procedures for the protection of subjects; mechanisms for obtaining informed consent; and the tasks of independent review committees.

- In 1989 the Law Reform Commission of Canada published Working Paper 61, entitled *Biomedical Experimentation Involving Human Subjects*. This Working Paper made a number of specific recommendations for the legal treatment of many of the important ethical issues raised by biomedical experimentation, including research on children and research involving the mentally ill.

- In 1990 the MRC adopted Guidelines for Research on Somatic Cell Gene Therapy in Humans. One of the Conclusions is that "Any attempt to treat an inherited disease by somatic cell gene therapy should be regarded as a research protocol, and subject to procedures and considerations as outlined in [the document] and in the MRC's *Guidelines on Research Involving Human Subjects*".

- The Canadian Medical Association's Code of Ethics, as revised in April 1990, includes a section on clinical research. It is specified that "an ethical physician... will ensure that, before initiating clinical research involving humans, such research is appraised scientifically and ethically and approved by a responsible committee and is sufficiently planned and supervised that the individuals are unlikely to suffer any harm. The physician will ascertain that previous research and the purpose of the experiment justify this additional method of investigation. Before proceeding, the physician will obtain the consent of all involved persons or their agents, and will proceed only after explaining the purpose of the clinical investigation and any possible health hazard that can be reasonably foreseen".

Chile. It appears that committees on medical ethics were established by Supreme Decree No. 446 of 29 December 1989. Details of the functions, etc. of these committees, notably as regards research on human subjects and community-based research, were laid down by Circular 2C/14 of 5 March 1990 of the Sub-Secretary for Health of the Ministry of Health. A number of texts are specifically endorsed, including Helsinki II and the 1983 Declaration of the Latin American Association of Academies of Ethics in Medicine (unavailable to the authors). The criteria to be employed by committees in reviewing research protocols from the ethical standpoint are formulated in detail.

Colombia. Sec. 54 of Law No. 23 of 18 February 1981 promulgating norms on the subject of medical ethics requires physicians to adhere to the recommendations of the World Medical Association in biomedical research in general and in therapeutic research (as specified).

Costa Rica. Article 5 of the Code of Medical Ethics of the College of Physicians and Surgeons of Costa Rica, adopted on 4 April 1981, requires physicians to adhere to the ethical principles of (*inter alia*) the Declaration of Helsinki.

Ecuador. The Revised Code of Medical Ethics of the Ecuadorian Medical Federation, dated 30 November 1989, includes a Chapter XX dealing with research and the updating of medical knowledge. Article 119 requires the physician to cooperate in scientific research on health, as well as in the development of new technologies and methods for the protection, restoration, and rehabilitation of patients. Under Article 120, research and experimentation on human subjects may only be performed by qualified physicians who comply with established ethical and scientific principles, the written consent of the experimental subjects being mandatory.

El Salvador. Certain provisions concerning experimentation are contained in the February 1986 Code of Medical Ethics issued by the Association of Physicians [*Colegio Médico*].

Guatemala. Chapter IV of Decree No. 0559 of 22 February 1991, which deals with various aspects of the prevention, control, etc. of HIV/AIDS, lays down that, in the absence of any specific legal provisions, therapeutic research on human subjects, particularly in respect of AIDS cases, is required to conform to the Declaration of Helsinki.

Haiti. It has been reported that a National Ethical Committee is being established, with the task of giving critical consideration to the ethical and legal issues raised by proposed studies involving human subjects.

Mexico. On 23 December 1986 the Secretariat for Health issued Regulations for the implementation of the General Law on health (of 26 December 1983), in the field of health research. Title II of these Regulations deals with the ethical aspects of research on human subjects. This Title is subdivided into the following Chapters: I. Joint provisions applicable to all categories of research; II. Research at the community level; III. Research involving minors or incompetent persons; IV. Research on women of child-bearing age, pregnant women, women during labour or childbirth, nursing mothers, and neonates; and on the use of embryos, stillborn and live fetuses, and assisted fertilization; V. Research on subordinate groups; and VI. Research on organs, tissues and their derivatives, products derived from human beings, and cadavers. Title III is entitled "Research on new prophylactic, diagnostic, therapeutic, and rehabilitative methods". The Mexican Regulations are among the most detailed in the developing countries.

Panama. Article 48 of the 1988 Code of Ethics of the National Medical Association of the Republic of Panama specifically endorses the recommendations of the World Medical Association concerning various topics, including biomedical research. One of the Notes to the Article lays down that a physician may not participate in any scientific research that is contrary to the will of any person.

Suriname. The Medical Investigations Approval Decree of 16 June 1981 lays down that medical research may be performed on groups of persons only with the prior approval of the Director of Public Health;

the conditions under which the research may be conducted are determined by the Director.

United States of America. Perhaps the most significant development during the decade was the issuance on 18 June 1991, by the Office of Science and Technology Policy of the Executive Office of the President, of a common Federal Policy for the Protection of Human Subjects (Model Policy), designed to achieve consistency in the regulations on this subject adopted by 16 departments and agencies of the Federal Government (it should be mentioned that the Central Intelligence Agency is required by an Executive Order to comply with the guidelines issued by the Department of Health and Human Services (HHS)). The provisions dealing with research in foreign countries are likely to be of considerable interest and read substantially as follows:

> ... This policy does not affect any foreign laws or regulations which may otherwise be applicable and which provide additional protections to human subjects of research.

> ... When research covered by this policy takes place in foreign countries, procedures normally followed in the foreign countries to protect human subjects may differ from those set forth in this policy. [An example is a foreign institution which complies with the World Medical Assembly Declaration (Declaration of Helsinki amended 1989) issued either by sovereign states or by an organization whose function for the protection of human research subjects is internationally recognized.] In these circumstances, if a department or agency head determines that the procedures prescribed by the institution afford protections that are at least equivalent to those provided in this policy, the department or agency head may approve the substitution of the foreign procedures in lieu of the procedural requirements provided in this policy.

- The basic HHS regulations for the protection of human subjects are contained in Part 46 (Protection of Human Subjects) of Title 45 (Public Welfare) of the United States Code of Federal Regulations. Prior to March 1983, Part 46 comprised the following subparts: basic HHS policy for the protection of human research subjects; additional protections pertaining to research, development, and related activities involving fetuses, pregnant women, and human in vitro fertilization; and additional protections pertaining to biomedical and behavioral research involving prisoners as subjects. In March 1983 the Federal Government amended Part 46 to provide additional protections for children involved as subjects in research. The new subpart distinguishes between: (1) research not involving greater than minimal risk; (2) research involving greater than minimal risk but presenting the prospect of

144

direct benefit to the individual subjects; (3) research involving greater than minimal risk and no prospect of direct benefit to individual subjects, but likely to yield generalizable knowledge about the subject's disorder or condition; and (4) research not otherwise approvable which presents an opportunity to understand, prevent, or alleviate a serious problem affecting the health or welfare of children. Also discussed are the requirements for obtaining the permission of parents or guardians and the assent of children.

- On 29 July 1983 additional provisions were inserted into Part 219 (Protection of Human Subjects in Department of Defense-Supported Research) of Title 32 (National Defense) proscribing the use of prisoners of war as subjects of research.

- With regard to embryo and fetal research, the Health Research Extension Act of 1985 (Public Law 99-158) provided for the insertion in the Public Health Service Act of a new Sec. 498 (Fetal Research) that reads as follows:

(a) The Secretary [of Health and Human Services] may not conduct or support any research or experimentation, in the United States or in any other country, on a nonviable living human fetus ex utero or a living human fetus ex utero for whom viability has not been ascertained unless the research or experimentation;

(1) may enhance the well-being or meet the health needs of the fetus or enhance the probability of its survival to viability; or

(2) will pose no added risk of suffering, injury, or death to the fetus and the purpose of the research or experimentation is the development of important biomedical knowledge which cannot be obtained by other means.

At the time of preparation of this paper, the status of this Section was uncertain.

- As an example of State legislation may be cited a California statute (Chapter 979 of 1989), which amended the State's Penal Code in the light of the consideration set forth in Sec. 1, as follows:

(a) The Legislature finds that state law designed to protect prisoners from inappropriate medical experimentation has had the unintended effect of preventing prisoners from having access to drugs or treatments which might be required for good medical care.

(b) The Legislature further finds that while the standard of practice for health providers practicing outside prisons has sometimes included access to "investigational new drugs" which the United States Food and Drug Administration allows to be made available for a serious or immediately life-threatening disease condition in patients

for whom no comparable or satisfactory alternative drug or therapy is available, health providers caring for state prisoners with HIV disease cannot use such drugs, even when they are determined to be the best medical treatment available to a particular prisoner.

(c) Therefore, it is the intent of the Legislature by this act to provide prisoners access to certain investigational drugs or treatments on the same basis that they are made available to patients outside the prison setting.

(d) It is the further intent of the Legislature to encourage ongoing evaluation of the effect that this section has on prisoners' medical care, particularly as it concerns people with AIDS or other forms of HIV disease, by requiring that affirmative steps be taken if the validity of this act is to extent beyond six years.

- The 1992 edition of the *Code of Medical Ethics: Current Opinions* of the American Medical Association's Council on Ethical and Judicial Affairs includes: guidelines intended to aid physicians in fulfilling their ethical responsibilities when they engage in the clinical investigation of new drugs and procedures; guidelines when undertaking clinical investigation primarily for treatment; guidelines when undertaking clinical investigation primarily for the accumulation of scientific knowledge; guidelines when conducting experimental or clinical investigation, such as with mechanical devices or animal organs, for the replacement of human organs that are no longer functional; and fetal research guidelines (with separate guidance for various kinds of fetal research).

- The January-April 1991 edition of *IRB: A Review of Human Subjects Research* (published by the Hastings Center, Briarcliff Manor, New York) includes an important paper by C. Levine, N. Neveloff Dubler and R.J. Levine entitled "Building a new consensus: ethical principles and policies for clinical research on HIV/AIDS". Following an introduction outlining basic concepts, existing mechanisms in the USA for accessing experimental drugs, and the US regulatory system, the article goes on to present 57 "Consensus Statements" (with accompanying commentaries), developed by a working group composed of experts in the field. On the specific subject of HIV/AIDS research, reference should also be made to a 1987 document entitled "Guidance for Institutional Review Boards for AIDS studies", issued by the Office for Protection from Research Risks of the National Institutes of Health. No information is available on the current status of this document.

- On 8 April 1992 the Public Health Service announced a final policy to make promising investigational drugs for AIDS and other HIV-related diseases more widely available under so-called "parallel track" protocols, while the controlled clinical trials essential to establish the safety and effectiveness of new drugs are carried out. This initiative establishes an administrative system designed to expand the availability of promising investigational agents, and to make them more widely available to people with AIDS and other HIV-related diseases who have no therapeutic alternatives and who cannot participate in controlled clinical trials.

Venezuela. There are detailed provisions on the clinical aspects of research on human subjects in Chapter 4 of Title V of the Code of Medical Ethics approved on 29 March 1985 in the course of the LXXVI Extraordinary Meeting of the Assembly of the Venezuelan Medical Federation.

The European Region

Bulgaria. Sec. 29 (2) of the Constitution of the Republic of Bulgaria, adopted on 12 July 1991, lays down that "no person shall be subjected to any medical, scientific, or other experimentation without his voluntary written consent" (a provision that is clearly derived from Article 7 of the International Covenant on Civil and Political Rights).

Czech and Slovak Federal Republic. Law No. 548 of 5 December 1991 of the Czech National Council amended Law No. 20 of 17 March 1966 on the protection of public health, notably by the introduction of a Sec. 27*b* prescribing, *inter alia*, that "the verification of new data on living subjects involving methods not hitherto used in clinical practice may only be carried out with the written consent of the person concerned as well as the written consent of the Ministry of Health". Prior to granting consent, the person concerned must be duly informed of the nature of the procedure, the way in which it is to be implemented, its duration, the objectives of the method, and the risks connected therewith. The verification of data as provided for above may not be performed on persons under detention or who have been deprived of their freedom, or on persons undertaking their basic military service, a "substitute service", or a civil service. There are further provisions in Sec. 27*c* dealing with medical procedures that do not present a direct benefit to the person involved (these are subject to the prior written consent of the person).

Denmark. Sec. 1 of Law No. 353 of 3 June 1987 provided for the establishment of an Ethical Council responsible for, *inter alia*, biomedical research involving human subjects. This Council is to work in cooperation with the health authorities and the scientific-ethical committees established in accordance with the Declaration of Helsinki. Other Sections of the Law require the Council to submit recommendations to the Minister of the Interior on certain categories of research.

- On 1 November 1988, the Minister of Health appointed a special Commission to examine whether "statutory provisions should be introduced in Denmark to regulate biomedical research involving live human subjects". The Commission's 111-page report, *Research Involving Human Subjects: Ethics/Law*, was issued in 1989. Among other aspects, it discusses the pros and cons of special legislation on this subject, and includes the text of a model bill.

- Important provisions on consent procedures in experimental projects are laid down in Chapter 2 of Circular No. 70 of 17 May 1991 defining physicians' duties and patients' rights. It is specified, in particular, that the normal requirements governing the duty of physicians to provide information and the manner in which consent is obtained are to be tightened whenever patients or healthy research subjects are involved in experiments (including clinical trials of medicaments). The information is to be given to the patient or healthy research subject both verbally and in writing.

- The 1990 Report of the Central Scientific-Ethical Committee of Denmark contains a series of Recommendations on research on human subjects. Recommendation No. 1 (October 1982, revised March 1986) deals with the requirements of informed consent; No. 4 (March 1984) with Danish biomedical research projects in developing countries (such projects are required to comply with Helsinki II); No. 5 (December 1983) with criteria for biomedical research on deceased persons; No. 6 (August 1984) with the use of research subjects who are employees of the pharmaceutical industry; No. 7 (October 1986) with research on patients "whose bodies function in a manner similar to that of healthy research subjects"; No. 11 (December 1987) with the payment of compensation to research subjects; and No. 14 (undated) with scientific research on mentally ill persons.

Finland. On 3 July 1985 the National Board of Health issued Circular No. 1987 concerning clinical trials of medicaments involving human subjects. This Circular includes the following rubrics: consent of experimental subjects; ethical evaluation of the experimental protocol; and insurance. The Circular specifically endorses the Declaration of Helsinki.

France. Certainly the most important development during the decade was the promulgation of Law No. 88-1138 of 20 December 1988 on the protection of persons participating in biomedical research. The effect of this Law (which was amended by Law No. 90-86 of 23 January 1990) was to insert a new Book II *bis* in the Public Health Code, subdivided into the following Titles: I. General provisions; II. Consent; III. Administrative provisions; IV. Provisions specifically applicable to research having no therapeutic objective; V. Penalties;

and VI. Miscellaneous provisions. Other provisions dealing with human experimentation were inserted in Book V (Pharmacy). A series of implementing decrees, ministerial orders, and circulars was issued subsequently, and includes: a Decree (No. 91-440 of 14 May 1991) on insurance coverage for sponsors of biomedical research; an Order (dated 28 December 1990) on the maximum amount of compensation payable annually to persons participating in biomedical research with no direct benefit to the individual; an Order (dated 14 February 1991) on the form to be used for declaring serious adverse effects liable to have been caused by biomedical research on a medicament or on a product placed on the same footing; a Circular (dated 1 October 1990) on the setting up of Advisory Committees for the Protection of Persons in Biomedical Research; and a Circular (dated 24 October 1990) on the role of care establishments in the protection of persons participating in biomedical research.[5]

- The legislation referred to above was preceded by an extensive debate in different circles and by the publication of a number of significant reports, notably *De l'Ethique au Droit* (1988), the outcome of a study undertaken by a Working Group chaired by M. Guy Braibant, President of the Reporting and Studies Section of the *Conseil d'Etat*. The Group had been set up by the *Conseil d'Etat* in response to a letter signed by the Prime Minister and dated 19 December 1986. The *travaux préparatoires* for the Law indicate the influence of the Working Group study, as well as of earlier reports and statements issued by the National Council of the Association of Physicians and the National Ethical Consultative Committee for the Life and Health Sciences (C.C.N.E.). The *travaux préparatoires* also refer to other international texts, including the Nuremberg Code, Helsinki II, and the WHO/CIOMS Proposed International Guidelines (referred to as the "Declaration of Manila").

- The new Law has already aroused considerable interest and some controversy. One of the proponents of the Law, Senator Claude Huriet, has recently published an article explaining its origins and history.[6] The International Association for Law, Ethics and Science (the so-called Milazzo Group) convened a colloquium (Paris, 21 November 1991) on the committee structures set up by the Law.[7]

- Several of the Opinions [*avis*] issued by the C.C.N.E. have dealt with various aspects of biomedical research, including research on human subjects. These have included the following: the Opinion of 9 October 1984 on ethical problems raised by trials of new therapeutic procedures; the Opinion of 24 February 1986 on patients in a chronic vegetative state (the use of such patients for experimental purposes is rejected); the Opinion of 15 December 1986 on *in vitro* research on human embryos and their use for

149

medical and scientific purposes; the Opinion of 17 November 1988 on ethical review committees; the Opinion of 2 December 1991 containing general reflections on the ethical problems posed by research on the human genome.

- An Instruction of 26 May 1987 of the Ministry of Defence refers to the Council on Medical Deontology of the Armed Forces and the Ethical Committee of the Armed Forces Health Service (C.E.S.S.A.). The latter body is responsible for giving its opinion to the Minister of Defence on non-therapeutic human experimentation conducted under the responsibility or with the participation of officers of the Armed Forces Health Service. It is, in particular, to examine deontological and ethical problems that may arise in cognitive research having no immediate and direct benefit for the experimental subject.

Germany. In a Notice dated 9 December 1987, the Federal Minister for Youth, Family Affairs, Women and Health issued Basic Principles for the Conduct of Clinical Trials of Medicaments. The objectives of these Principles are stated as:

1.3 Before a clinical trial is initiated, its ethical and legal bases should be examined. The criteria are the provisions of clinical trials laid down in Sections 40 and 41 of the Medicaments Law [of 24 August 1976] and the Declaration of Helsinki (as amended in 1983). An independent and competent ethical review committee should be consulted.

1.4 Persons planning or conducting clinical trials should bear in mind that a balance must be struck between the duty of care owed to the individual patient or experimental subject and the general desire for therapeutic progress. The risks for participants in tests must be medically justifiable in relation to the anticipated importance of the medicament for medical science.

As an example of other provisions contained in the Basic Principles, the following criteria are laid down for trials involving pregnant or breast-feeding women:

3.2 Clinical trials during pregnancy or breast-feeding should only be conducted if:

3.2.1 the medicament is intended for protection against, or the diagnosis, treatment, or alleviation of, diseases suffered by pregnant or breast-feeding women or by unborn children;

3.2.2 according to the present state of medical knowledge, the use of the medicament is indicated in the case of pregnant or breast-feeding women or of unborn children, in order to diagnose diseases or their evolution, to treat or alleviate diseases, or to protect the pregnant or breast-feeding woman and the unborn child;

3.2.3 according to the present state of medical knowledge, no unjustifiable risk for the unborn child should be anticipated in the conduct of the clinical trial; and

3.2.4 the clinical trial, according to the present state of medical knowledge, cannot be anticipated to yield adequate results unless it is carried out on pregnant or breast-feeding women.

- On research on human embryos, the Federal Chamber of Physicians adopted *Guidelines for Research on Early Embryos* on 4 October 1985. Among other provisions, these Guidelines proscribe research on human embryos if: (1) it could be performed on animals; (2) it does not serve any immediate or medium-term prophylactic, diagnostic, or therapeutic purpose; or (3) it does not comply with rigorous scientific and procedural standards. The Guidelines go on to specify that the use of human embryos for research purposes requires the informed consent of the genetic parents. Other restrictions relate to the *in vitro* development of embryos, cloning, the creation of chimeras, and interspecific hybridization. Detailed provisions concerning various procedures on human embryos (some of which are no doubt research procedures) are contained in the Embryo Protection Law of 13 December 1990.

Hungary. Provisions concerning research on human subjects are contained in Ordinance No. 11 of 19 August 1987 of the Minister of Health on biomedical research; this is to some extent based on the provisions of Helsinki III. Sec. 7, which relates to informed consent, reads as follows:

7. (1) A biomedical intervention may be undertaken on a patient or on a person in good health who voluntarily and freely consents to undergo experimentation. Any biomedical intervention [of this nature] is subject to the prior written consent of the research subject. In the case of a person whose competence is limited, the consent of the research subject and that of his legal representative are both required. In the case of a person under 14 years of age, consent shall be given by his legal representative.

(2) Persons whose competence is limited and persons above 14 years of age but who are totally incompetent may be the subject of biomedical interventions for therapeutic purposes that are directly associated with their disease or state of health.

(3) Minors may be involved in biomedical interventions only for purposes of the prevention, diagnosis, or treatment of diseases occurring in children or for rehabilitation purposes.

(4) Biomedical interventions may not be undertaken on persons who:

(a) are not Hungarian citizens;

(b) are in preliminary detention; or

(c) are serving a sentence of imprisonment in a penitentiary establishment.

Ireland. In 1986 Guidelines relevant to the Procedure for Conduct of Clinical Trials were issued by the National Drugs Advisory Board of Ireland. They include a discussion of the role, composition, etc. of ethical committees, the informed consent of participants in clinical studies, and "problem areas for informed consent".

Israel. In September 1989 the Pharmaceutical Administration of the Ministry of Health issued a document entitled "Procedure for the Submission of an Application for Approval of a Clinical Trial in a Hospital, in accordance with the Public Health (Medical Experiments Involving Human Subjects) Regulations, 1980". Among other provisions, it is laid down that such applications are to be submitted to the hospital's Helsinki Committee; if approved, the application is thereafter forwarded to the Ministry of Health in Jerusalem. It is indicated that the text of the "patient's informed consent" must include a full and clear explanation of the trial, its objective, and the risks involved therein. There must likewise be a written commitment by the manufacturer/importer to supply the medicament in question without charge.

Italy. Clause 3 of Bill No. 5563 of 21 March 1991 promulgating new rules governing clinical trials on human subjects lays down that (1) trials may not be conducted on healthy minors, mental patients, criminal detainees, political detainees, prisoners of war, or persons whose freedom of movement has been restricted, on societal or other grounds, nor may any remuneration be paid to experimental subjects; (2) certain phases of clinical trials, as specified, may be conducted on pregnant women, neonates, and minors suffering from diseases, subject to specific assurances concerning any possible risks; (3) a patient always has the right to the most effective treatment possible and to respect for his person, in precedence over any other interest; and (4) the patient's consent must be given in writing (in the case of a minor suffering from a disease, the consent is given by the minor's legal representative). No information is available as to the current status of this Bill.

- There are evidently provisions on the ethical aspects of clinical research in the 1989 revision of the Code of Medical Ethics (unavailable to WHO).

- A Ministerial Decree of 27 April 1992 laid down provisions dealing with the technical documentation to be attached to applications for a marketing authorization for medicinal products for human use, in conformity with Commission Directive 91/507/EEC of 19 July 1991. This lays down, *inter alia*, that the ethical standards contained in the Note for Guidance on Good Clinical Practice for Trials on Medicinal Products in the European Community (GCP), developed by the CPMP (Committee for Proprietary Medicinal Products) Working Party on Efficacy of Medicinal Products, must be adhered to insofar as the ethical aspects of experimentation on human subjects are concerned; the GCP guideline was completed in July 1990, and had an implementation date of 1 July 1991.

- An example of legislation at the subnational level is Regional Law No. 46 of 30 August 1982 of Umbria, Sec. 4 of which provides that: (1) trials must be performed with respect for the individual; (2) trials must not prejudice any citizen's right to health, or make any distinction between citizens with regard to that right; (3) the patient's free, informed consent must be obtained in advance; and (4) specific trials (e.g. for tolerance, safety, efficacy, etc.) require the approval of the Regional Technical Health Council.

Luxembourg. Provisions concerning human experimentation are contained in Secs. 26-28 of the Code of Ethics of the Medical and Dental Professions, approved by an Order of 21 May 1991 of the Minister of Health. Sec. 27 requires experimental protocols to be submitted in advance to an independent ethical committee, while under Sec. 28 the experimental subject's free and informed consent is required (a potential experimental subject must be informed of his right not to participate in the experimentation and to withdraw therefrom at any time).

Netherlands. In 1982 the Central Public Health Council published a Partial Report on Medical Experiments Involving Humans, one of a series of reports issued after the publication of a 1978 report on patients' rights. It provides a brief survey of relevant legislation in the Netherlands and in other countries, followed by a discussion of the requirements to be fulfilled for experiments involving human subjects, with particular reference to ethical review committees. A draft law on medical experiments is under consideration by the Ministry of Health, Welfare and Cultural Affairs. It provides for the establishment of a Central Committee on Medical Experimentation, with both administrative and substantive responsibilities; that body would replace the existing Interim Central Committee on Ethical Aspects of Medical Research.

Norway and Sweden. Highly relevant information on the functioning of research ethics committees in these two countries is presented in a recent paper by Solbakk.[8] As regards Norway, in 1983 the Medical Research Council issued Ethical Guidelines on Research in Children, while in 1987 the same body issued guidance on information and consent in biomedical research. In 1990, guidance on research on fetuses was issued jointly by the Council and the Norwegian General Scientific Research Council.

Poland. The new Code of Medical Ethics, adopted on 14 December 1991 in the course of the II Extraordinary National Congress of Physicians, includes a chapter entitled "Scientific research and medical experimentation", comprising Secs. 43-52. Sec. 43 lays down that biomedical experiments performed by physicians on human subjects must conform to the generally accepted principles of scientific research. Under Sec. 44, any experimental project involving human subjects must be clearly formulated in writing, and be evaluated by an independent ethical review committee for purposes of approval. Under Sec. 47, the experimental subject must be duly informed of all aspects of the experiment and may at any time suspend his participation. A person consenting to participate in an experiment must not be influenced by the physician. Sec. 48 deals with experimental subjects who are incapable of giving their consent.

Spain. The most recent item of legislation at the national level on the ethical aspects of human experimentation is Law No. 25/1990 of 20 December 1990 on medicaments. Title 3 of this Law is entitled "Clinical trials", and consists of a single chapter, comprising Secs. 56-69. Sec. 60 (Compliance with ethical principles) is substantially reproduced below:

> *60. All trials shall be subject to the administrative authorization laid down in Section 65, and, in addition, the following requirements shall be met:*
>
> *1. ...*
>
> *2. clinical trials shall be conducted under conditions which respect fundamental human rights and the ethical principles relating to biomedical research in which human beings are involved, the contents of the Declaration of Helsinki and the successive Declarations updating these Principles being complied with for this purpose;*
>
> *3. ...*
>
> *4. it shall be necessary to have the freely expressed consent, preferably in writing or, failing this, before witnesses, of the person on whom the trial is to be conducted, after such person has been informed by the health professional in charge of the research as to the nature, significance, scope, and risks of the trial and after having understood that information;*

5. in the case of clinical trials without any particular therapeutic interest for the experimental subject, consent shall always be given in writing;

6.-7. ...

Sec. 62 deals with insurance coverage, while Sec. 63 indicates the responsibilities of the sponsor, person in charge [monitor], and principal investigator. Under Sec. 64 no clinical trial may be undertaken without a prior report by an ethical committee on clinical research, which must be independent of sponsors and investigators and have been duly accredited by the competent health authority (which must have given notice thereof to the Ministry of Health and Consumer Affairs). Details are given of the principles that must govern the work of such committees, and their composition (they must consist of an interdisciplinary team made up of physicians, hospital pharmacists, clinical pharmacologists, nursing personnel, and persons outside the health professions, including at least one lawyer). Detailed provisions on administrative interventions in respect of clinical trials are laid down in Sec. 65, while Sec. 66 deals with the methods of clinical trials. Provisions for the financing of trials are laid down in Sec. 67. Under Sec. 69 (Publications) the results of various clinical trials are to be published in scientific journals, with the name of the ethical committee that issued a report on the trial. It is understood that this Law has repealed Crown Decree No. 944/1978 of 14 April 1978 on clinical trials involving human subjects, and the Order of 3 August 1992 for its implementation.

• There are detailed provisions concerning research on human embryos and fetuses and their biological structures in Chapter III of Law No. 42/1988 of 28 December 1988 on the donation and use of human embryos and fetuses or their cells, tissues, or organs. Thus, Sec. 7 reads as follows:

7. (1) Basic research on human embryos and fetuses or their biological structures shall be authorized only if it is in compliance with the provisions of this Law and is based on duly formulated protocols that have been examined, and, where appropriate, approved by the public authorities responsible for health and scientific affairs, or, if so delegated, by the National Commission for Supervision and Control of the donation and utilization of human embryos and fetuses.

(2) The teams responsible for research and/or experimentation shall communicate the results to the authorities which approved the corresponding protocol either directly, or in cases where this is required by regulations, through the National Commission for Supervision and Control.

– **Basque Autonomous Community**. The Charter of Rights and Obligations of Patients and Users of the Basque Health Service, approved by Decree No. 175/1989 of 18 July 1989, includes provisions on patients' and users' rights with regard to research, such as the "right to refuse to be the subject of health research", and the "right not to undergo diagnostic or therapeutic procedures if their effectiveness has not been established".

Switzerland. On 17 November 1981 the Swiss Academy of Medical Sciences issued revised Guidelines for Experimental Research on Human Subjects. On 11 May 1989 the Academy issued revised Guidelines for the organization and activities of medical-ethics committees responsible for reviewing projects for medical experimentation on human subjects. These include sections on: the protection of data relating to experimental subjects; insurance coverage for experimental subjects; and medical research elsewhere than in hospitals.

- There is no Federal legislation on human experimentation, but a number of cantons have issued statutory or regulatory texts on the subject. Thus, Sonnabry *et al.* report that nine of the cantons have a law that regulates ambulatory and institutionalized clinical research, while in six other cantons clinical research in hospitals is regulated by secondary legislation (the 11 remaining cantons have no legislation on this subject).[9] In the Canton of Berne the Decree of 14 February 1989 on patients lays down that physicians are not entitled to involve their patients in research without their express consent. They are required to do so in compliance with the Academy's Guidelines, if the Executive Council declares them to be applicable; Sec. 1 of the Ordinance of 14 November 1989 on experimental research in human subjects lays down that the Guidelines are in fact applicable, and must be complied with in all experimental research. There are somewhat similar provisions in the Law of 6 December 1987 of the Canton of Geneva on relationships between members of the health professions and patients. In the Canton of Jura the Health Law of 14 December 1990 lays down, in Sec. 30, that no clinical trial may be undertaken without the consent of the persons concerned. If a person lacks the capacity of discernment, a clinical trial may be undertaken only if its objective is to bring about a beneficial effect on that person's state of health. The Guidelines are specifically endorsed in Sec. 45 of the Health Law of 20 October 1991 of the Canton of Obwald and in Sec. 9 of the Patients' Ordinance of 28 August 1991 of the Canton of Zurich. The Canton of Ticino has detailed provisions on human experimentation in Secs. 10-13 of the Health Law of 18 April 1989.

United Kingdom. The position in the United Kingdom is rather complex, given that there is no statutory legislation on the subject (other than provisions of limited scope in the Human Fertilisation and Embryology Act 1990 — see *infra*), and the significant number of bodies and organizations that have been active in the field. As pointed out in a Press Notice issued in May 1986, the Medical Research Council (MRC) published a detailed statement entitled "Responsibility in Investigations on Human Subjects" nearly 25 years ago (which originally appeared in the MRC's Report for 1962-63). The MRC has pointed out that the statement remains in force (although it is currently under review). The guidance it provides has been incorporated into advice issued subsequently by the Royal College of Physicians of London (RCP). The MRC's position on informed consent and other key ethical issues has been stated as follows:

> *In general, the patients participating in them should be told frankly that different procedures are being assessed and their co-operation invited. Occasionally, however, to do so is contra-indicated. For example, to awaken patients with a possibly fatal illness to the existence of doubts about effective treatment may not always be in their best interest.*

> *The progress of medical knowledge has depended, and will continue to depend, in no small measure upon the confidence which the public has in those who carry out investigations on human subjects, be these healthy or sick. Only in so far as it is known that such investigations are submitted to the highest ethical scrutiny and self-discipline will this confidence be maintained. Mistaken, or misunderstood, investigations could do incalculable harm to medical progress. It is our collective duty as a profession to see that this does not happen and so to continue to deserve the confidence that we now enjoy.*

In 1985 the MRC issued *Responsibilities in the Use of Personal Medical Information for Research: Principles and Guide to Practice*; and a statement entitled *Research Related to Human Fertilisation and Embryology* (this statement may have been superseded by the 1990 Act).

- During the last few years the RCP has issued a number of significant reports on research on human subjects. These include its 1986 report, *Research on Healthy Volunteers*; the 2nd Edition of *Guidelines on the Practice of Ethics Committees in Research Involving Human Subjects* (1990); a 1990 report, *Research Involving Patients*; and the 1991 report, *Fraud and Misconduct in Medical Research: Causes, Investigation and Prevention*. Owing to space constraints it is not possible in this paper to explore these in any detail. Suffice it to say that they are critical for understanding how research on human subjects is, as it were, "self-regulated" by the medical profession in the United Kingdom.

- In 1991 the Department of Health issued a publication entitled *Local Research Ethics Committees*. In particular it discusses the role of the National Health Service (NHS) in enabling medical research to be conducted. Details are given of the NHS bodies that are expected to refer to LRECs for advice on the ethics of proposed research projects. It specifies, *inter alia*, that an LREC must be consulted about any research proposal involving: NHS patients; fetal material and *in vitro* fertilization involving NHS patients; the recently dead, on NHS premises; access to the records of past or present NHS patients; and the use of, or potential access to, NHS premises or facilities.

- The British Medical Association's *Handbook of Medical Ethics* (1984) contains a section on "Research in human subjects". This points out, *inter alia*, that "Codes, regulations and laws help to keep standards of ethical behaviour high, but volunteers and patients are best protected by ethical conduct. The subjects' interests must come first". Reference is made to the Declaration of Helsinki. There are sections on research on children, on prisoners, and in occupational medicine. In 1988 the *Handbook* was issued in revised form as *Philosophy and Practice of Medical Ethics*. This reproduces the full text of Helsinki III, thereby implicitly endorsing its provisions, as far as members of the BMA are concerned.

- The Association of the British Pharmaceutical Industry has issued a series of texts relating to human experimentation. The July 1989 *Guidelines for Medical Experiments in Non-Patient Human Volunteers* replaced previous Guidelines issued in 1970 and 1984. *Guidelines on Good Clinical Research Practice* (May 1988) addressed, *inter alia*, ethical review by independent ethics committees and informed consent procedures, and included a 15-point listing of the "elements of informed consent". On 7 November 1990 the Association issued *Guidelines for Ethical Approval of Human Pharmacology Studies Carried Out by Pharmaceutical Companies*, as well as *Guidelines for Research Ethics Committees Considering Studies Conducted in Healthy Volunteers by Pharmaceutical Companies*; and in July 1991 it issued *Guidelines on Clinical Trials — Compensation for Medicine-Induced Injuries*, which has the status of a recommendation by the Association to its member companies.

- The Medical Sterile Products Association issued in 1986 *Guidelines for the Design and Conduct of Clinical Trials for Medical Devices*, which includes sections on considerations prior to the initiation of clinical trials; the organization of clinical trials; patient confidentiality; clinical trials in countries other than the United Kingdom; and record-keeping. There is a series of appendices, one of which describes briefly requirements in France, the Federal Republic of Germany, Japan, the United Kingdom, and the United States of America for the conduct of clinical trials of medical devices.

- Mention should be made of the Code of Practice on the Use of Fetuses and Fetal Material in Research and Treatment, derived from the Review of the Guidance on the Research Use of Fetuses and Fetal Material (the so-called "Polkinghorne Report"), published in 1989.

- Sec. 11 of the Human Fertilisation and Embryology Act 1990 establishes a system of licensing of research on human embryos. Under the terms of paragraph 3 of Schedule 2 to the Act, such licences may be granted for any of the following (for the purposes of a research project specified in the licence): bringing about the creation of embryos *in vitro*; and keeping or using embryos. However, a licence may not authorize any research activity unless it appears to the Human Fertilisation and Embryology Authority to be necessary or desirable for the purpose of promoting advances in the treatment of infertility; increasing knowledge about the causes of congenital disease; increasing knowledge about the causes of miscarriages; developing more effective techniques of contraception; developing methods for detecting the presence of gene or chromosome abnormalities in embryos before implantation; or such other purposes as may be specified in regulations made under the Act.

- In 1991 the Scottish Law Commission issued a Discussion Paper, *Mentally Disabled Adults: Legal Arrangements for Managing Their Welfare and Finances.* A recent summary of this Paper notes: "The legality of carrying out non-therapeutic medical research on people who lack mental capacity is doubtful. The Commission proposes that non-therapeutic research on mentally incapable subjects should be permitted only if: it is in connection with the subject's mental disability, it has been approved by the appropriate Ethics Committee, it poses minimal risks to participants, written consent has been given by the subject's nearest relative or personal guardian, and the subject does not object".[10]

- In 1991 the Medical Research Council issued a series of three reports dealing with various aspects of medical research. These were: *The Ethical Conduct of Research on Children; The Ethical Conduct of Research on the Mentally Incapacitated;* and *The Ethical Conduct of AIDS Vaccine Trials.*

159

- In January 1992 the Committee on the Ethics of Gene Therapy (which the Government had set up on 28 November 1989) submitted its Report to Parliament. The "Summary of Main Conclusions and Recommendations" addresses the ethical basis of gene therapy, stating that "gene therapy should initially be regarded as research involving human subjects". Gene therapy should therefore "conform with accepted ethical codes whose purposes, together with the means of giving them force, are to: (a) facilitate justifiable advancement of biomedical knowledge; (b) maintain ethical standards of practice; (c) protect the subjects of research from harm; (d) preserve subjects' rights and liberties; and (e) provide reassurance to the public, to the professions and to Parliament that these are being done". The Report considers which aspects of gene therapy research are justifiable, and the conditions that should be met for such research to be ethical and seen to be so. There are detailed discussions on (1) somatic-cell gene therapy, and (2) germ-line gene therapy (it is recommended that "gene modification of the germ line should not yet be attempted"). Another section deals with the supervision of gene therapy, and it is recommended that a "supervisory body with the necessary collective expertise, experience and authority be set up, having the responsibility for making [the relevant] assessments in conjunction with local research ethics committees". Details are given of the recommendations regarding the areas of responsibility of this supervisory body. The final section deals with "Control and discipline". One of the recommendations is that "gene therapy be confined to a small number of centres whilst experience is gained".

- In June 1992 the British Paediatric Association issued revised Guidelines for the Ethical Conduct of Medical Research Involving Children, to replace its 1980 Guidelines on the subject.

- In the spring of 1992 a private organization, the King's Fund Institute, issued a report, *Ethics and Health Care: The Role of Research Ethics Committees in the United Kingdom*. It includes significant conclusions and a range of detailed recommendations on such issues as the constitution and working of research ethics committees, consent and other ethical issues, and policy issues (with particular reference to research design, financial issues, legal liability, enforcement and sanctions, and studies undertaken by general practitioners). The "major recommendation" of the report is that there should be "legislation to strengthen [the role of research ethics committees], and to empower them to carry out their genuine tasks properly, with the support and training they require".

160

Libyan Arab Jamahiriya. Law No. 28 of 3 November 1986 concerning medical responsibility includes provisions laying down that no scientific experiment may be performed on a living person "except with his prior consent, and only for the realization of a desirable benefit to such person and with the knowledge of other physicians licensed to perform such experiments on the basis of recognized scientific principles".

Saudi Arabia. Ministerial Resolution No. 288/17/L of 23 January 1990 promulgates Rules for the implementation of the Regulations on the practice of medicine and dentistry, which prescribe that it is professional malpractice to conduct unapproved experiments or scientific research on a patient.

Tunisia. There are detailed provisions concerning the ethical aspects of research on human subjects in Decree No. 90-1401 of 3 December 1990 establishing the modalities for medical or scientific experimentation on medicaments intended for use in human medicine. Sec. 1 lays down that such experimentation must be undertaken "in accordance with the international conventions on health and human rights that have been ratified by Tunisia, and the rules of medical deontology and ethics that deal with human experimentation". Secs. 2-5 of the Decree are reproduced below:

> *2. Medical or scientific experimentation on medicaments intended for use in human medicine may be undertaken only on persons who have reached the age of majority and enjoy all their mental faculties and legal capacities.*
>
> *No experimentation may be performed on minors, mental patients, mentally handicapped persons, or on pregnant women or nursing mothers.*
>
> *By way of exemption from the preceding provisions, mental patients and mentally handicapped persons may be subjected to medical experimentation having therapeutic objectives that are specific to their disease or handicap. In such cases, the written consent of the guardian shall invariably be required.*
>
> *3. Medical or scientific experimentation on medicaments intended for use in human medicine shall be carried out without financial compensation or any other form of [corresponding] transaction.*
>
> *4. No medical or scientific experimentation may be performed on human subjects:*
> > *— unless it is based on the latest scientific knowledge, and on adequate experimentation on animals after* in vitro *studies; and*

— unless the foreseeable risk to persons participating in the experimentation is proportional to the anticipated benefit to such persons.

5. Before medical experimentation is performed on a human subject, his free, informed, and written consent must be obtained, after a clinical expert in charge of the trial has acquainted him with:
— the objective of the investigations, and their methodology and duration; and
— the constraints and foreseeable adverse effects.

The Western Pacific Region

Australia. In 1983 the National Health and Medical Research Council (NHMRC) adopted a Statement on Human Experimentation; it is accompanied by four Supplementary Notes, and was issued in the light of Helsinki II and the WHO/CIOMS Proposed International Guidelines. The Statement, which is "to be read in conjunction with the Supplementary Notes", deals with "[e]xperiments [that] range from those undertaken as a part of patient care to those undertaken either on patients or on healthy subjects for the purpose of contributing to knowledge, and include investigations on human behavior". Supplementary Note 1 deals with the functions and constitution of institutional ethics committees. Supplementary Note 2, adopted by the Council in 1982 and revised in 1987, deals with the ethics of research on children, the mentally ill, and those in dependent relationships. Supplementary Note 3 deals with therapeutic trials, and Supplementary Note 4 with *in vitro* fertilization and embryo transfer. In 1988 the NHMRC republished the Statement, with three additional Supplementary Notes. Supplementary Note 5 discusses research involving human fetuses and human fetal tissue; Supplementary Note 6 is a statement on the conduct of epidemiological research; and Supplementary Note 7 deals with somatic-cell gene therapy.

- In 1987 the NHMRC endorsed a report on Ethical Aspects of Research on Human Gene Therapy; interesting perspectives on this issue are contained in the NHMRC's report on a Round Table Conference on Gene Therapy held on 2 September 1988.

- The Privacy Act of 1988 includes provisions authorizing the NHMRC, with the approval of the Privacy Commissioner, to issue guidelines for the protection of privacy in the conduct of medical research involving humans. These guidelines are not examined here, since they fall outside the overall purview of this article.

- In 1991 the NHMRC issued a report entitled *Guidelines for the Use of Genetic Registers in Medical Research*. They addressed such issues as approval and consent procedures, the responsibility of

162

"Keepers" of genetic registers, and the responsibilities of institutional ethics committees.

China. On 2 February 1988 the Ministry of Public Health issued Rules governing the approval of clinical trials of foreign drugs. Under Sec. 9 of these Rules, clinical institutions are required to closely monitor experimental subjects in the course of clinical trials, and ensure their safety.

Hong Kong. Hong Kong is one of the jurisdictions that have incorporated into their domestic laws certain provisions of the International Covenant on Civil and Political Rights. Thus, Article 3 of the Hong Kong Bill of Rights Ordinance 1991 lays down, *inter alia*, that "no one shall be subjected without his free consent to medical or scientific experimentation".

Japan. Provisions dealing with the ethical review of research on human subjects (including healthy subjects) are contained in Notification No. 874 of October 1989 of the Pharmaceutical Bureau of the Ministry of Health and Welfare, on "Good Clinical Practice (GCP) for Trials of Drugs", which entered into force in October 1990.[11]

New Zealand. Sec. 10 of the New Zealand Bill of Rights Act 1990 echoes Article 7 of the International Covenant on Civil and Political Rights, in laying down that "every person has a right not to be subjected to medical or scientific experimentation without that person's consent".

- Sec. 18(1)(*f*) of the Protection of Personal and Property Rights Act 1988 lays down that no court may empower a welfare guardian, and no welfare guardian of an incapacitated person has the power, "to consent to that person's taking part in any medical experiment other than one to be conducted for the purpose of saving that person's life or of preventing serious damage to the person's health".

- The 1989 New Zealand Medical Association Code of Ethics includes a section that deals with clinical research (it is stated that this section "summarizes the principles outlined in the Declaration of Helsinki"). Reference should also be made to Sec. 24 of the Health Research Council Act 1990, which established an Ethics Committee. A substantial amount of information on these and other recent developments is contained in David B. Collins' *Medical Law in New Zealand*, published in 1991.

Philippines. On 1 April 1982 the Office of the Minister of Health issued an Administrative Order on Research Policies and Guidelines in the Ministry of Health. Sec. 4 of Part III (Guidelines for Research

Involving Human Subjects) includes the following provisions on community-based research:

> *... informed consent is not necessary where community-based research is to be undertaken, such as the experimental treatment of water supplies, or trials of new insecticidal, prophylactic, or immunizing agents, nutritional adjuvants or substitutes, etc., although it is essential that the community, and in particular its leader, be fully informed of the study. Dissenting individuals should have the option not to participate. The decision for community participation rests upon the responsible health authority of the community.*

These provisions are clearly based on the corresponding provisions in the 1982 WHO/CIOMS Proposed International Guidelines.

Conclusions

From this paper it is clear that there has been considerable international, national, and subnational regulatory activity in the field of human experimentation during the decade under review. However, as Jayasuriya[12] has noted, many developing countries still lack an appropriate legislative, regulatory, or administrative framework. Meanwhile many of the industrialized countries have greatly enlarged the scope of regulation in this field, to include areas that were scarcely on the agenda at the time of the Manila Conference in 1981. Much remains to be done, not least in the light of the continuing debate on, for example, the ethical aspects of experimentation on new medicaments for the treatment of AIDS,[13] and on more critical, far-reaching issues, in developing countries in particular.

Notes and References

1. Fluss, S.S. The proposed guidelines as reflected in legislation. In: Bankowski, Z. & Howard-Jones, N., Eds. *Human Experimentation and Medical Ethics* (Proceedings of the XVth CIOMS Round Table Conference, Manila, 13-16 September 1981). Geneva, CIOMS, 1982, pp. 323-366.
2. For a very helpful and perceptive compilation of papers on diverse aspects of human experimentation and epidemiological research, see Dickens, B.M., Gostin, L. & Levine, R.J., Eds. Research on human populations: national and international ethical guidelines. *Law, Medicine & Health Care*, 19(3-4): 157-295 (1991). For perspectives on historical and current issues, see Annas, G.J. & Grodin, M.A., Eds. *The Nazi Doctors and the Nuremberg Code: Human Rights in Human Experimentation*. New York and Oxford, Oxford University Press, 1992.
3. See in this connection Perley, S. et al. The Nuremberg Code: an international overview. In: *The Nazi Doctors and the Nuremberg Code: Human Rights in Human Experimentation, supra* ref. 2, at pp. 135-160.
4. These Guidelines have been published in the following sources: Bankowski, Z., Bryant, J.H. & Last, J.M., Eds. *Ethics and Epidemiology: International Guidelines* (Proceedings of the XXVth CIOMS Conference, Geneva, 7-9 November 1990). Geneva, CIOMS, 1991; *Law, Medicine & Health Care, supra* ref. 2, at pp. 247-258; and *International Digest of Health Legislation* 1992; 43(1): 180-198. The Proceedings volume includes a contribution (at pp. 76-91), which may be regarded as

complementary to the present paper, viz. Fluss, S.S., Simon, F. & Gutteridge, F. *Development of international ethical guidelines for epidemiological research and practice: a survey of policies and laws.*

5. In September 1991 the French Ministry of Social Affairs and Integration issued a two-volume compilation of all the relevant legislative, regulatory, and international texts on this subject, as well as a guide thereto. Readers desiring background information on the developments that led to the new French legislation should consult S. Gromb's doctoral thesis on "*La recherche biomédicale sur l'être humain face au droit français*" (presented to the University of Bordeaux I in 1992). A noteworthy earlier French doctoral thesis is J. Duclaux's "*L'expérimentation du nouveau médicament sur l'homme: étude de droit comparé*" (presented in 1985 at the National School of Public Health in Rennes).

6. *International Digest of Health Legislation* 1992; 43(2): 391-93.

7. See the article by C. Byk in *ibid.*, 393-97.

8. Solbakk, J.H. *HEC Forum* 1991; 3(4): 215-220.

9. *Médecine et Hygiène*. 1992; 50: 113-34. Reference should also be made to the comprehensive inventory of Swiss Cantonal legislation on research on human subjects, compiled by Sprumont, and to the doctoral thesis presented by Ummel to the Faculty of Medicine of the University of Geneva in 1991 on the subject "*La réglementation de l'expérimentation humaine et l'organisation des commissions d'éthique médicale en Suisse*". Sprumont's compilation has been heavily drawn upon in the preparation of the section on Switzerland.

10. *Commonwealth Law Bulletin* 1992; 18(1)_ 181-83.

11. *Japan Medical News*, April 1990, Special Issue, pp. 2-4.

12. Jayasuriya, D.C. Law, ethics, and biomedical research involving human subjects in developing countries. *Journal of Clinical Research and Drug Development* 1989; 3: 83-88.

13. Byar, D.P. *et al.* Design considerations for AIDS trials. *New England Journal of Medicine* 1990; 323: 1343-47.

Acknowledgements

The authors wish to thank the numerous persons and institutions who contributed information and materials used in the preparation of this paper. In particular they acknowledge the contributions of: F. Simon and D.L. Heymann (WHO, Geneva), H.L. Fuenzalida, D.S. LaVertu, and A.M. Linares (WHO Regional Office for the Americas/Pan American Health Organization, Washington, DC), M. Barbu (Geneva), J. Donovan (Canberra), E. Faupel (Geneva), R.H. Nicholson (London), J.H. Solbakk (Oslo), D. Sprumont (Fribourg), and F.O. Wells (London). The secretarial support of Mrs Marilyn Vogel and Ms Christine Raynor was unstinting and invaluable.

A special word of thanks goes to Dr Zbigniew Bankowski, Secretary-General of CIOMS, for his strong encouragement and support of this study.

Note

To keep the size of this paper to reasonable limits, the authors have not given references for the great majority of laws, regulations, codes, etc. cited. Virtually all of these have been or are due to be reported in the WHO quarterly journal, *International Digest of Health Legislation*. Except where clearly indicated, all translations are unofficial. The authors alone are responsible for any errors, omissions or misinterpretations, to which they would appreciate their attention being drawn.

AN ANNOTATED GUIDE TO ETHICAL REVIEW OF RESEARCH INVOLVING HUMAN SUBJECTS

Lawrence Gostin* and Lisae Jordan*

In 1989, when the decision was taken to revise and update the CIOMS Proposed International Guidelines for Biomedical Research Involving Human Subjects (1982), it was decided to develop, as a separate publication, International Guidelines for Ethical Review of Epidemiological Studies, which was published in 1991, and also An Annotated Guide for Ethical Review of Research Proposals, to be used as a practical tool to help in applying the various existing international ethical guidelines. This paper summarizes the purposes and contents of the Annotated Guide.

The Annotated Guide is intended for the use of investigators, ethical review committees, and others concerned with research involving human subjects, to help them understand clearly and make the best use of ethical guidelines. It is directed to a broad audience in both developing and developed countries: clinical and epidemiological researchers, sponsors of research, those who appoint ethical review committees, members of ethical review committees, teachers and students of public health, and ministries of health and other government agencies concerned with the ethical implications of research in their countries.

Purposes of the Annotated Guide

The Annotated Guide to Ethical Review is intended to provide a systematic bridge between the various international ethical guidelines on human-subject research and the practical needs of those conducting such research. It is not meant to replace international guidelines. It is a second-level document, highlighting the principles of established guidelines and outlining pertinent issues for discussion.

The ethical issues discussed in the Annotated Guide are derived from primary and secondary source materials. The most important primary sources are the Nuremberg Code, the Declaration of Helsinki, the CIOMS International Guidelines for Ethical Review of Epidemiological Studies, and the CIOMS International Ethical Guidelines for Biomedical Research Involving Human Subjects.

The secondary source materials relied on in the Annotated Guide are regional or national guidelines; they include the Council of

---

* American Society of Law & Medicine, Boston, Massachusetts, U.S.A.

Editorial note: The draft Annotated Guide has been used in the preparation of the revised guidelines and for their annotation.

Europe's Recommendation to Member States concerning medical research on human beings, issued in 1990; the Recommendations on Human Subject Research by the Law Commission of Canada, issued in 1989; and, from the United States, The Belmont Report: Ethical Principles and Guidelines for the Protection of Human Subjects of Research, issued by The National Commission for the Protection of Human Subjects of Biomedical and Behavioral Research, in 1978.

Critically well-received books and articles on biomedical research comprise the final level of source materials; they are used to explain and amplify the ethical principles. They provide useful sources for further exploration by researchers and ethical review committees as well as for continuing education and training.

The Annotated Guide will present in a question-and-answer format the legal, ethical and practical issues associated with each international ethical guideline.

The Guide has also an educational purpose — the study of ethical issues in human subject research; it includes a bibliography to encourage more in-depth examination of the issues.

Many countries do not have sufficient human and financial resources for adequate ethical review, but the establishment of a capacity for such review should be a high priority. The Annotated Guide is intended to be of use to national authorities in developing this capacity.

Aids to Ethical Review

The Annotated Guide contains three parts: (i) an annotated checklist, (ii) an abbreviated checklist, and (iii) a model memorandum of understanding.

Each is divided into the same twelve basic sections: scientific considerations, risk-benefit evaluation, subject selection, consent, community consensus, confidentiality, health care provided for human subjects, compensation for accidental injury, the relationship between sponsoring countries and host countries in international collaborative research, the building of an infrastructure and a capacity of ethical review in host developing countries, access to the benefits of research, and ethical review committees.

(i) The annotated checklist

Each of the twelve sections is organized according to guiding principles, questions, and answers. The guiding principles set out the ethical foundation for the guidelines. The guidelines on informed consent, for example, are derived from the ethical principle of respect for persons, which requires investigators to respect the autonomy of persons capable of self-determination, and to protect vulnerable subjects.

168

The guiding principle is followed by a series of legal, ethical and practical questions designed to help researchers and review committees apply ethical principles to the protocol in hand, systematically and thoroughly. Thus, with regard to informed consent, there are questions on each element of consent: legal capacity, comprehension, voluntariness, and adequacy of information. In this way researchers and ethical review committees can review each question, discuss it with their colleagues, and come to a decision as to whether the ethical responsibility has been fulfilled in that respect.

Often the questions suggest an answer, but do not require an explicit decision. Many ethical issues require a considered balancing of competing interests. For example, one ethical guideline refers to the protection of vulnerable subjects. Vulnerable subjects such as children should not usually be selected for research involving significant risks. This ethical guideline, however, can clash with the guideline requiring equity in subject selection. If vulnerable groups such as children, pregnant women, or institutionalized persons are systematically excluded from research, they cannot gain the benefits of the research, and the results of the study will not be generalizable to those groups. It is because researchers have often erred on the side of excluding vulnerable subjects that so little is known about how beneficial drugs and vaccines will affect the health of pregnant women and children.

Each series of questions is followed by a discussion designed to clarify the pertinent ethical issues. The questions on vulnerable subjects, for example, are clarified by a discussion of the several categories of people commonly considered vulnerable, such as children, prisoners, and persons with disabilities.

(ii) The abbreviated checklist

The abbreviated checklist of ethical and practical questions uses the same organization and the same set of questions as the annotated checklist, but without the annotations of guiding principles, discussion, and source materials. Once the Annotated Guide has been read and carefully used, researchers or committees may wish to use the simpler, shorter document on a routine basis, or they may decide to use the abbreviated checklist together with the annotated checklist, referring to the explanatory discussion only when they feel uncertain or want a fuller discussion.

Ethical issues may arise that are not on the checklist: the research may raise novel or unusual ethical problems; the application of research to local cultures and mores may require a different ethical emphasis; or it may be simply that the ethical questions faced have not been resolved in international guidelines. The questions posed in the checklist are designed to alert researchers and review committees to all the ethical issues that may arise in a research project.

(iii) A model memorandum of understanding

The model memorandum of understanding is intended for use by investigators engaged in international collaborative research. It covers the key areas where it is desirable to reach understanding between researchers from source and host countries in international collaborative research. Also, it may serve as a model for collaborative or multicentre research in a single country.

The model memorandum of understanding is not directive or intended to be a contract or legal instrument. Rather, it provides a framework within which researchers can come to an advance understanding about issues important to the sponsors, investigators and subjects of the research. This helps foster respect between researchers, which is increasingly recognized as ethically important. Strong collaborative relationships help develop human resources in the host country, and make future research projects more welcome and professional.

CULTURAL
PERSPECTIVES ON ETHICS AND
RESEARCH ON HUMAN SUBJECTS

AN AFRICAN PERSPECTIVE

B.O. Osuntokun*

I find it difficult to contribute to this session without repeating what
has been said on previous occasions, at this and earlier conferences
organized by CIOMS, notably the Athens Conference of 1984 on
Ethics and Human Values: An International Dialogue and the Geneva
Conference of 1990 on *Ethics and Epidemiology: International
Guidelines.* For example, in 1990 Abdussalam and Osuntokun stated
that, although the objectives of ethical review of all types of
biomedical research were universal, individual items of review had to
be adapted to conditions frequently met with in developing countries
and in the context of their sociocultural backgrounds. We then went
on to give examples of such items: unsuitable topics of study;
inappropriate conduct of studies; inadequate preparatory studies;
informed consent and cultural modifications that may be required in
applying the basic principles; externally-sponsored research; and
compensation for injury. We discussed also the need to set up ethical
review procedures in developing countries; to build up capacity for
ethical review; to disseminate and use results; and the desirability of
making available to communities in developing countries where
research such as vaccine trials has been carried out the benefits of
such research. Earlier at this conference, I discussed some of these
issues as they relate particularly to informed consent, against the
sociocultural background of communities in Africa.

Very briefly, the relevant cultural attitudes in Africa that may
influence applications of ethical guidelines include the following:

1. Concepts of disease and disease aetiology may differ from orthodox
   biomedical concepts. Many communities in Africa still believe in
   supernatural causes of disease, and find it difficult to accept that
   bacterial and viral infections cause disease states. More recently,
   especially with the serological testing for HIV antibodies becoming
   commonplace in some communities, seropositivity denoting the
   presence of antibodies after trials of vaccines may be unacceptable
   as it may be interpreted as being synonymous with disease.

2. Some communities in Africa, because of their religious beliefs, are
   unusually stoical and indifferent to suffering and pain. This may
   influence their tolerance and acceptance of harmful effects of
   research in relation to potential benefit. In some communities, even
   death may not be considered "harmful", as it is regarded as not the
   end of life, but as entry into another, usually better, life.

---

* Department of Medicine, University of Ibadan, Ibadan, Nigeria.

3. In some communities, there is strong societal influence on the concept of personhood, and an individual may be very willing to sublimate or sacrifice personal interests for the benefit of others.

4. In many parts of Africa, family ties and bonds are still very strong. A wife-and-husband relationship may be regarded as inseverable, but a wife may be denied legal competence in some communities.

5. Community leaders may constitute the most reliable, and in some communities the only, bridge to a community or society.

6. Many communities in Africa still have the highest respect for the physician, who is often regarded as omniscient, to be trusted at all times for decisions about health and disease. Such paternalistic and patronising relationships between patients or other prospective research-subjects and physicians will tend to make prospective subjects accept whatever proposals physicians make to them, and this could lead to exploitation and abuse.

7. Widespread illiteracy in most parts of Africa makes comprehension harder, but not impossible.

Abdussalam and Osuntokun (1990) concluded: "The peculiarities of the conditions of most Third World countries... place additional responsibilities on the shoulders of those who are to assure that unethical actions do not infringe the human rights of the individuals and communities in which biomedical and epidemiological studies are carried out. Nevertheless, we agree it would be naive to expect guidelines to be quickly and effectively absorbed or applicable in Third World countries, where poverty, severe underdevelopment and illiteracy are pervasive. Guidelines, however, are not regulations, but there is need for minimum floor guidelines to assure a level of observance of ethical standards below which no one should fall".

However, it is necessary to re-emphasize two important points that are relevant to the perspective of the African with regard to ethical guidelines and research: (i) the changing nature of the culture of the African, and (ii) the recent severe socioeconomic decline. These have implications for ethical guidelines and research.

There is enormous diversity in the culture and characteristics of the peoples of Africa, although there are also some commonalities. The Hamites in North Africa, the West African Negroes in the West, and the Bantu Negroes in East, Central and Southern Africa differ in many respects in their indigenous cultures. However, two of the monotheistic religions commonly referred to as the Abrahamic religions (Judaism, Christianity and Islam), namely Islam and Christianity, are widely embraced in the continent; even the third, Judaism, has its practitioners among the Falashis of Ethiopia (who were recently air-lifted *en masse* to the State of Israel). For example, in Nigeria about

45% of the 120 million inhabitants (a quarter of the population of Africa) are Muslims and an equal number are Christians. It has been suggested that the original impetus for modern bioethics in some Caucasian countries such as the United States of America came from religion-driven moralism. Religion has a strong influence on culture in Africa, and there are now only small proportions of the population who can be said to have retained undiluted the "original indigenous culture". In Nigeria, Christianity was established in some parts as far back as 1850 (the first Nigerian was enthroned as an Anglican Bishop in 1859) and Islam much earlier. Christianity fully supports research, for Jesus Christ said "Seek and ye shall find", and so does the Prophet Mohammed, who decreed that "the pursuit of knowledge is a mandate on every Muslim, man or woman" and taught his followers that the angels "lower their wings in respect for those who seek knowledge". The Quoran recommends the prayer "O my Lord, advance me in knowledge". It is relevant to state that all African states subscribe (at least on paper) to the concept that research is an essential tool for development. The Organization of African Unity, established in 1960 and now comprising all countries in the continent, in its charter exhorts member states to devote at least 1% of their gross domestic product (GDP) to research and development.

Apart from the influence of religion, people in Africa are increasingly becoming better educated and more amenable to change. Since 1960 the political wind of change has created a new sense of awareness of self. It should therefore not be too difficult for the researcher to comply with basic ethical principles (with the appropriate modification to cope with cultural sensitivities) that regulate research involving human subjects.

The current socioeconomic milieu in Africa is relevant to some bioethical issues. The economies of most African countries have deteriorated over the last decade, with negative or only small annual economic growth, huge national debts, crippling repayment rates of national debts, with several countries paying interest charges in excess of their foreign-exchange earnings. Most of the countries allocate less than 2% of gross domestic product to health-care services. A good number are devastated by wars (some lasting for the past two decades or more), drought, failed agricultural policies and hence widespread poverty and malnutrition, explosive population growth and brain drain. In some countries in sub-Saharan Africa the health of the population is now worse than it was a decade ago. Only about 50% of the countries have mechanisms for managing health-related research and for control of ethical issues in health care and health-related research.

The greatest medical ethical need in most of the African countries is justice and equity in allocation of resources and distribution of effective health-care services. This must be borne in mind in determining research priorities and in collaboration with external sponsors of research to be carried out in recipient countries in Africa. While I agree that it is not the function of an ethical committee to determine national research priorities, nevertheless it should have some discretion in pointing out gross anomalies, such as the absurdity of conducting research on frost-bite on the banks of the river Niger!

Cultures have unique explicit and implicit beliefs about the values that should inform and govern personal and communal life. These are bound to influence the practice and application of ethical guidelines in biomedical research involving human beings. For example, Judaism has serious reservations about autopsy, which for the physician is a critical procedure for gaining further understanding of disease. Roman Catholics would frown at, or even totally reject, experiments on artificial fertility control. Islam emphasizes the will of Allah. Some "indigenous" Africans would deny legal competence to a wife. As stated earlier, in some cultures diseases are believed to have supernatural origin; among some communities, death is the end of life, while in others it is the entrance to another, usually better, life. I believe that we must appreciate and respect differences in the cultures of people, and understand the need to use, if necessary, different approaches and a great deal of ingenuity to achieve our objectives in research involving human beings — that is, the observance and practice of good ethics and good science. I fully concur with the view that ethical requirements for performing biomedical research involving human subjects in Third World countries may be more, rather than less, exacting and taxing than in the developed countries.

Let me end on a humorous note, on the need for universal respect for persons and the dignity of humans. A community may have a very distinguished background of history and culture. I as a Yoruba from Nigeria have very many close friends of all races. One particularly distinguished one from Wales used to joyfully torment me that I was a savage, even though a happy one. I was always delighted to riposte after the manner of Disraeli, the famous British Prime Minister of the latter part of the 19th century, that my ancestors came from Egypt and the Middle East, and that the predecessors of my distinguished friend lived in caves under the colonial yoke of the Romans centuries after mine had already been glorious priests in the courts of the Pharaohs.

ASIAN PERSPECTIVES:
VACCINE TRIALS IN THAILAND

N. Bahmarapravati*

My presentation deals with practical ethical matters in the conduct of trials of a live attenuated dengue viral vaccine in my own country, Thailand. It has been an instructive experience of trying to harmonize a trial of dengue vaccine, a product of science and technology, with the culture, traditions, values and beliefs of an Asian society.

A unique feature of the trial is that the vaccine was developed in Thailand, not transferred from an industrialized country to be tested in the usual way in a developing country. From both procedural and ethical viewpoints the experience has taught us that, in a developing country, to be able to apply ethical principles to biomedical research requires a fair level of infrastructure and technology.

Dengue vaccine trials raise several ethical issues. The plan calls for the development of monovalent vaccines for each of the four serotypes of the viruses. The trials for safety and immunogenicity will be conducted for the four monovalent vaccines, then for the three bivalent vaccines, then for a trivalent vaccine and finally for a tetravalent vaccine. Infection with one type of dengue virus results in the development of an antibody for that type, but the individual risks becoming seriously ill if infected after a certain interval with another type of dengue virus. Vaccination with a monovalent vaccine carries the same risk. There is therefore an ethical problem, which we hope is partially avoided by performing the trials of dengue vaccines in places far away from urban communities, where the transmitting vector, *Aedes aegypti*, is not found, and from where the vaccinated individuals are very unlikely to come to towns or cities and be bitten by the *Aedes aegypti* mosquito. The trial site is over 700 km from Bangkok.

A major problem was our lack of people familiar with the procedures for the approval of clinical trials with regard to human experimentation. Three groups in particular are concerned: the investigators, the reviewers or referees concerned with human experimentation, and the volunteers for vaccination.

The investigators

The scientific rationale for safety of the products normally rests on reports of the safety of the vaccines in animals, as well as on an impartial review by the national food and drug administration through the initial procedure for reviewing a new drug. Since for dengue there is no animal model, there are no safety data from animal tests. As an assurance of safety we have followed fully the requirements of the U.S.

---

* President, Mahidol University, Bangkok, Thailand.

Food and Drug Administration for a live attenuated viral vaccine; these requirements include a neurovirulence test in monkeys as well. There is no Thai FDA. The World Health Organization, which has been supporting the programme for the past 12 years, has appointed an international peer committee to review the scientific and technical performance of the vaccine development project, and it was this committee that advised WHO and the Thai Ministry of Public Health that the vaccines were ready for human trial. This experience testifies to the conditions of a developing country and to the possibility of devising alternative means of fulfilling safety requirements. Whether these means satisfy ethical requirements others may judge differently.

The Experimentation Committee of the Ministry of Public Health

Although one would expect that this committee would be well-informed about the international ethical guidelines for research on human subjects enunciated in the Declaration of Helsinki, it appeared not to be. Its members have not been selected on the basis of interest in, or knowledge of, ethical procedures relating to human experimentation. There have been several changes of chairman in the six years of its existence, and each has been Director-General of the Department of Medical Service. The appointment of the Director-General to chair this committee may indicate the importance that the Ministry of Public Health accords to ethical review of human experimentation, but the Director-General is a very busy person, with a heavy load of activities and obligations.

Moreover, the holder of this post is changed every one to two years, which prevents continuity and tends to block any dynamism in the refinement of procedures or processes on the basis of experience. The committee has been sometimes lenient and sometimes, on irrational matters, very harsh. Also, though this vaccine trial is unique and innovative in many ways, no member of the committee has ever expressed a wish to make an observational or site visit to the trial. It has been satisfied merely to review the process and procedures by going through the papers and questioning the investigators. This raises questions of seriousness of intent and the extent to which a developing-country authority has mastered ethical review procedures.

The volunteers for vaccination

In a developing country, communities and social groups differ greatly in their levels of knowledge and information, and in this respect the trial volunteers are considered to be at the bottom of the hierarchy of Thai communities. The need to use remote communities may be responsible for this. Though we applied carefully and most conscientiously the concept of informed consent, and consent forms were duly signed, we could not satisfy ourselves that we had complied

178

fully with the international guidelines. We attribute this to the very low level of general knowledge or understanding of scientific and technical information on the part of the volunteers and their communities.

The exercise of individual freedom and choice is complicated by the fact that in Thailand, beyond an individual's biological instinct of survival, there is the notion of social sensitivity, which Westerners like to call "face-saving". If there is no risk of bodily harm or social disgrace, the vaccine trials appear to be acceptable to many in the community. The allegation that scientists from industrialized countries are using "human guinea-pigs", sometimes made in regard to other trials, stems from the mistaken notion that somehow participation in a vaccine trial involves loss of face more than risk of harm. The fatalistic approach to life should make it easier to recruit volunteers, but the loss of face associated with being confined to a clinic or hospital for observation and daily physical examination and recording of body temperature has made recruitment more difficult. It has been difficult also to persuade volunteers to return to give blood samples or to be interviewed after six months or a year. Another factor to be considered is poverty, which makes the giving of money, gifts, or services to volunteers a very delicate matter. In addition to reimbursement of expenses, volunteers may be compensated for loss of daily earnings during confinement in hospital after immunization. Ten dollars a day for three weeks of observation and daily blood-drawing may seem a fortune to a villager who must travel for three hours by car on a dirt road to reach a highway almost 800 km from Bangkok. The notion of adequately informing volunteers to enable them to judge freely and to choose to give "informed consent" seems irrelevant in these circumstances.

After a couple of the trials were conducted, and to satisfy ourselves that we had observed fully the principle of informed consent, we began informally to solicit informed consent of "peers" of the volunteers in addition to that of the volunteers themselves. These "peers" were some respected elders of the families or communities of the volunteers, and included venerable Buddhist monks, village headmen, and school-teachers, among others.

The assessment of the efficacy of dengue vaccine in the trial depends to a certain extent on the behaviour of the volunteers — in minimizing travel to towns where they risk being bitten by *Aedes aegypti* and getting a natural infection of dengue, which would interfere with the pattern of antibody response from vaccination. The honorarium they were given induced a number of them to visit the town, some for the first time.

For other vaccines, such as a HIV vaccine, the risk factor connected with behaviour of relatively uneducated people with a fatalistic approach to life may be an ethical problem. Such people may have false confidence in the efficacy of a HIV vaccine and therefore increase their own risks by more adventurous sexual behaviour. The use of placebo in this kind of trial may also be unethical as it may lead to false confidence among some recipients.

* * *

Ethics is an important element of Asian culture, tradition, values and beliefs. In Northern and South-East Asia, where Chinese culture is influential, the ethics of the everyday activities of individuals and families may be very important. In Western and South Asia, the ethics may be expressed in the woven fabric of religious precepts and, at times, mysticism. The former group may find it easier than the latter group to conceptualize an ethical approach to human experimentation. In general, and although ethics is important and intricately woven into the traditional society, modernization does not bridge well with traditional ethics. This is true of modern science and technology as well as of other professions. Asian societies may have to find ways to look at modernization through their own cultures, values and beliefs rather than through Western ethics, and try to apply those alien principles in their own societies. The harmonization of ethical principles with the application of science and technology appears to be an evolutionary process difficult to achieve in the short term. Yet the moulding of ethical principles with the modernization of developing countries and their traditional societies could be crucial to the successful outcome of development itself.

ASIAN PERSPECTIVES: EXPERIMENTATION ON HUMAN SUBJECTS IN JAPAN — BIOETHICAL PERSPECTIVES IN A CULTURAL CONTEXT

Rihito Kimura*

Introduction: cultural background

The phrase *jintai jikken* (human experimentation) is taboo in the Japanese sociocultural context. Experimentation on other human beings, sometimes even on animals, is regarded as cruel, degrading and not acceptable in both Confucian and Buddhist thought, nurtured in the Japanese traditional religion of Shintoism.

Almost all Japanese medical schools hold special ceremonies at least once a year in memory of all animals experimented upon and killed for research purposes. Many researchers are expected to attend this *ireisai* (memorial service) according to Shinto or Buddhist tradition. The Japanese had to accept scientific experimentation in medicine and biology for the sake of research and development. This was in contrast to the Japanese sense of attachment to animal beings.

Humans are regarded as part of all living beings and acts of loving-kindness to all fellow living-beings are a very important virtue in the Japanese cultural tradition. This is therefore part of the character of medical practice. The preface of the first Japanese medical encyclo-pedia, entitled *Ishinpo*, edited by Yasuyori Tamba in 30 volumes and published in 982 A.D., states that such "medical service is the expression of the great mercy of Buddha and the loving-kindness of Confucian teaching".

Traditionally accepted standards of medication, practice and treatment, which originated in China, have been well developed and dominant in Japan. Western medicine, particularly the German medical model, came to Japan only at the end of the last century, when Japan engaged in its modernization process.

Although in Japanese traditional medicine generally there is reluctance to perform human experimentation, there have been some exceptions. An example is the case of breast-cancer surgery in 1805, in which general anaesthesia was used for the first time in medical history. Dr Seishu Hanaoka (1760-1835) used his new combination of traditional herbal medicine on his mother and his wife for the validity and efficiency test, and finally for the successful operation of breast cancer.

Traditional Confucian teaching stated "Do no harm to one's body, which was given by one's parents, since this is the source of filial piety". However, in the Japanese cultural context, when the situation

---

* Professor, School of Human Sciences, Waseda University, Tokorozawa, Japan; Kennedy Institute of Ethics, Georgetown University, Washington, D.C., U.S.A.

was very critical and it was important to help and serve others, as in the case of Dr Hanaoka with his research trial, his wife and even his mother were willing to submit themselves to a justified experimental procedure as an expression of their affection for their husband and son. Internal family relationships and psychological elements in the sociocultural background of Japanese society at the beginning of the 18th century were beautifully analysed in the novel, *The Wife of Seishu Hanaoka*, written in 1966 by one of Japan's most eminent female novelists. Particularly in rural communities, the family unit and family bonds are expected to be very strong and easily recognizable.

Live organ donations among family members, even in the experimental stages, are common because of these familial ties. It is a unique aspect of Japanese organ transplantation that 70% of kidney donations are from living donors, and in all cases of segmental liver transplantation the donation is from one of the recipient's parents. This is because brain-death criteria have not been established for cadaver organ donation in Japan.

Japanese sentiment nurtured in traditional culture still survives in every sphere of life, even in westernized medical settings. For the general public, it is simply impossible to accept a dualistic approach to mind and body, to the notion of brain-based human personality, and to the technical replacement of human body parts in experimentation on human beings.

Behind this reluctant attitude of the Japanese public to experimental medical technology have been various symbolic medical tragedies that have come to public attention recently. Recovery of trust in medicine and in the medical profession is the key to demystifying the phrase *jintai jikken*, mentioned at the beginning of this paper.

Patients as research material — "the Dr Wada incident"

It is essential in medical experimentation on human subjects that there should be strict conditions to protect the rights of the patients. Without having final applications of all kinds of technological inventions and medications in the treatment and cure of disease, new developments in medical science would not be realized.

In Japan, as I mentioned briefly before, the general public has not been seriously aware of the importance and meaning of *jintai jikken*, and has simply rejected the idea of human experimentation. Medical professionals and researchers were seriously mistrusted and thought to be insincere. This is a reasonable and acceptable reaction from the lay public's point of view, as there have been several reports of cases clearly categorized as *jintai jikken* (human experimentation).

Such a typical case was "the Dr Wada incident". This happened in 1968, when Dr Wada became the first Japanese surgeon to perform a human heart transplantation. This was only the fourth transplantation in the world. The heart was taken from a drowning victim and transplanted to a patient with heart failure from mitral stenosis and insufficiency. The recipient died after 83 days and Dr Wada's disclosures about both the donor's and the recipient's clinical data aroused serious suspicions. These doubts involved his brain-death criteria decision, his lack of an alternative treatment suggestion without having obtained full informed consent from the families of both the patient and the "donor", and a rather hasty transplantation without having done sufficient basic research beforehand on such problems as graft rejection or postoperative infectious disease.

Dr Wada was accused of wrongdoing and this led to criminal investigation by the Sapporo District Attorney's Office, although he was not indicted. In 1970 a public gathering was held in Tokyo on the issues raised by the Dr Wada incident. "The Declaration of Patients' Rights" was officially announced at the end of the meeting. Its contents were very simple in proclaiming the protection of the rights of patients, with special reference to the Dr Wada incident. Now, 24 years later, many people still remember this, and Dr Wada still insists that he did nothing wrong.

It is quite true that until very recently the physician's unquestioned paternalistic authority was an accepted reality of Japanese medical culture. It is accepted practice to perform therapeutic research or to do research on patients in the name of clinical trial, in closed confidential clinical settings, usually without full informed and written consent, and with no peer review before or after treatment. There has been no public scrutiny and there is little tendency to malpractice litigation (the average number of new malpractice cases is around 400 a year) as the Japanese public traditionally have a very strong sense of respect, trust and obedience with regard to physicians, without knowing the details of what is happening to their bodies.

The Dr Wada incident opened up the core issue of the physician-patient relationship. The incident was totally unbelievable because it broke the traditional "trust" relationship. The societal trauma of *jintai jikken* became a nightmare for many people by revealing the symbolic research-oriented mentality of advanced medical experts such as Dr Wada and others who dared to do *jintai jikken* on patients as mere research material.

The source of professional failure
in bioethics and ethics committees in Japan

Almost all "ethics committees" for biomedical research and innovative treatment in Japanese medical schools or hospitals have some guiding principles and bylaws, including some statements of policies, to guide ethical decision-making. These principles and policies always reflect the relevant accepted codes of standards and professional consensus on ethical principles in medical practice and research issued by international medical and health organizations, including the Council for International Organizations of Medical Sciences, the World Medical Association and the World Health Organization.

Public concern about the protection of the patient in therapeutic research and of research subjects was considerable at the time of the Dr Wada incident. However, an increasing number of *jintai jikken* have been reported by the mass media since the middle 1950s, but very few criminal charges have been brought against the medical researchers. Neither have there been any serious efforts to set up ethics committees in accordance with bioethical guidelines. In November 1984 for the first time in a Japanese medical school, the Tokushima University, officially established "The Ethics Committee", to review the research protocol of *in vitro* fertilization.

Japan has no national regulations requiring any sort of review committee such as the institutional review board in the USA. All 80 medical schools and some other hospitals voluntarily have their own local ethics committees. They usually claim to have guidelines for clinical research trials or therapeutic research in accordance with the Declaration of Helsinki and, in some cases, mention the CIOMS Proposed International Guidelines (1982).

CIOMS documents on ethics committees were particularly influential and became basic reference material for the ethics committee established in 1981 at the Tokyo University Institute of Medical Sciences.

Although Japanese medical researchers are becoming aware of international trends in protecting the rights of human subjects involved in clinical research, there seems to have been no serious internal or professional initiative reflecting disclosure in the actual *jintai jikken* mentioned above, when setting up ethics committees.

During World War II, war crimes committed by Japanese military medical professionals in Northern China at Unit 731 were not taken seriously as the outcome of a systematically structured problem of the Japanese medical community. Rather it was noted as an exceptional case, due to the extraordinary war-time situation. Several cases of actual *jintai jikken* were performed with human "material", mainly on Chinese captives, to verify the results of research for the production of biochemical weapons, freezing experiments, bacterial infection experimentation, exposure to poison gas, etc.

Unlike the Nuremberg Trial defendants, all of the Japanese medical criminals were granted immunity from punishment for their inhuman crime of experimentation on captives, in exchange for giving all "extraordinarily valuable" data to U.S. Army researchers. Forty years after these secret deals, by using the Freedom of Information Act of the U.S. Federal Government, I investigated some of the "top secret" documents of the U.S. Occupation Forces and the Pentagon, kept at the National Records Center in Suitland, Maryland. It was considered "a matter of national security" not to give any resource material or information to Communist countries by opening up the issues of the Tokyo War Tribunal. This superseded the matter of justice and prosecution of medical professionals. I feel that we missed the timely chance of total disclosure, immediately after the war, of this very serious crime of human experimentation by Japanese medical experts in China. If the Japanese medical community had had in place a similar code of medical ethics as that which followed the Nuremberg trials, the Japanese public would have trusted the medical community.

Other experiments on humans, which resulted in the death of human subjects, were performed in China and even in Japan on captives of the allied forces. These were done in the name of vivisection practice and for the collection of some anatomical data. The vivisection case, which happened at the Kyushu University Medical School, was brought to the Yokohama War Crimes Tribunal. The record clearly shows the violation of international law, as well as the war-time mentality of the medical professionals in seizing all possible chances to perform medical research.

New trends regarding *rinsho chiken* (clinical trial)

The pace of development of bioethical ideas is slow. However, the medical professional community cannot now function without social support, including the support of the lay public.

In 1986 the Japan Medical Association set up its Bioethics Council, composed of 10 members from other professions, including the legal, the social-anthropological, the business, the philosophical, and the biochemical fields, as well as the medical profession. Bioethical topics chosen by this Council were "Brain death and organ transplantation", "Pre-sex selection of the fetus", "Care of the terminally ill patient" and "Explanation and consent". In the final report, issued in January 1992, the Japan Medical Association, one of the most authoritative Japanese medical organizations, for the first time endorsed the notion of the "Japanese way" of informed consent being applied in the clinical and research setting. The *setsumei* (explanation) by the physician to the patient and *doi* (consent) are strongly recommended. This is a considerable advance over the situation in the early 1980s when I began to challenge the Japanese medical profession to emphasize the bioethical aspects of medical services and patients' rights issues.

Now bioethical problems are so well reported in the Japanese daily newspapers that even the phrase "informed consent" has become common parlance not only among medical professionals but also among the lay public.

There have been no permanent bioethics commissions at the national level, but special bioethics boards, affiliated with the Ministry of Health and Welfare (*Koseisho*), have existed since 1983-85. During the two year-year period 1990-92, there was an Ad Hoc Commission on Brain Death and Organ Transplantation, which had been established under the Prime Minister's Office (*Sorifu*).

Because of the complication of the Dr Wada incident, many Japanese are reluctant to accept organ donations from cadavers diagnosed as brain-dead. The Japanese Federation of Diet Members on Bioethical Issues is preparing special legislation relating to organ transplantation in order to integrate existing legislation with that governing transplantation of kidneys and corneas.

In the case of the drug-testing protocol for prospective pharmaceutical products, the system of Good Clinical Practice (GCP) was initiated in 1990 by the Ministry of Health and Welfare. This is in accordance with international trends in procedural justification of research protocols, informed consent of subjects, and the constitution of ethical review committees.

In the face of extraordinarily rapid biomedical, biotechnological and pharmaceutical development, people in Japan feel that it is important to protect the weak and the sick, particularly children, women and the aged. Some of the Japanese lay public have taken the initiative in developing aspects of bioethics that focus on patients' rights. There is a movement to propose new legislation for the protection of patients' rights, for the family as well as for responsible health-care institutions, communities and government organizations.

Conclusion

In this age of the global community it would be naive to overemphasize the uniqueness of a particular cultural heritage in human, family and social relations. It is true that different cultural and ethical values should be respected, such as key concepts of the dignity of each human person, the importance of the family unit, and community life, but justification of any act or behaviour against human dignity and the rights of the person for the sake of cultural tradition is not acceptable.

In this sense we need international dialogue and understanding for the establishment of internationally acceptable guidelines for conducting research, especially biomedical research. In Japan we have learned much from the 1982 Proposed International Guidelines for Biomedical Research Involving Human Subjects (CIOMS) and it has been a challenge to our cultural tradition. Because of its impact, as well as public input from national and international sources, the situation of clinical and research setting is clearly changing.

The Japan Association for Bioethics was formed in 1988. There are now more than 20 bioethics-related projects in process and several research centres have been established. Since 1987 compulsory bioethics courses have been required at the School of Human Sciences of Waseda University for all 600 senior students. Human experimentation issues have been one of the main topics of these courses, which are jointly taught by three faculty members — a biologist, a medical scientist and a lawyer bioethicist (R.K.). Increasing the number of courses and curricula in bioethics studies at various levels of educational institutions would greatly increase awareness in Japanese society of medical-service and health-care issues.

The very recent amendment, in June 1992, to the Medical Service Act (1948) accepted the new provision that not only physicians but also nurses, pharmacists and other health-care workers are providers of medical services. Also, in the new supplementary provision, the notion of informed consent has been mentioned as a basis of trust between physician and patient. It states also that full implementation of this concept is a continuous task of the welfare and health administration for the preparation of a total amendment of the Act, possibly soon.

The issue of *jintai jikken* (human experimentation) will not be taboo any more in view of these new developments and expressions of concern about bioethical problems. As Japanese we are encouraged to be members of the global community by fully participating in the international process of developing ethical guidelines for biomedical research involving human subjects.

References

Kimura, Rihito, Ethics Committees for "High Tech" Innovations in Japan, *The Journal of Medicine and Philosophy* 1989; 14: 457-464.

Kimura, Rihito, Japan's Dilemma with the Definition of Death. *Kennedy Institute of Ethics Journal* 1991; 1: 123-131.

Kimura, Rihito, Fiduciary Relationship and the Medical Profession: A Japanese Point of View, In: E.D. Pellegrino et al. Eds. *Ethics, Trust, and the Professions: Philosophical and Cultural Aspects*, pp. 235-245. Georgetown University Press, Washington, D.C., 1991.

National Archives and Record Administration, U.S. Government, Gray File (Unit 731 Related Documents).

National Archives and Record Administration, U.S. Government, Documents on Trial, Aihara et al. (Yokohama Military Tribunal).

UNESCO, Bioethics and Human Rights. *Human Rights Teaching*, No. 4, Paris, 1992.

ASIAN PERSPECTIVES: TENSION BETWEEN MODERN VALUES AND CHINESE CULTURE

Ren-Zong Qiu*

I am often invited to discuss a subject from the Chinese perspective. Sometimes I ask myself what is meant by "Chinese" or what it refers to. As they become more integrated with the rest of the world, the Chinese become more diverse in their beliefs and values, from typical traditional Chinese to totally Western. Most, however, are intermediate, like me. In this paper I discuss the characteristic view of Chinese culture, the view of Chinese professionals, and my own view.

Modern or Western medicine in China was a transplant from the *manyi zhi bang* ('barbarian and alien countries'). It was not successful until the end of the 19th century; at that time European physicians successfully treated many high-ranking officials of the Qing Dynasty whom traditional doctors could not cure. The strategy of paying particular attention to high-ranking officials resulted in the acceptance and wide spread of Western medicine. In contrast, their 17th century predecessors, the Jesuits, had adopted an unsuccessful strategy: they lectured on Western scientific and medical theories to the Emperor, and he denounced them as *dia chong xiaoji* (insignificant skill). As Western medicine became dominant its traditional counterpart declined. Its theories and its clinical practices are well received in China, though such terms as *yin yang, qi* (vital energy), *xu* (deficiency), and *shang huo* (heat arises) are still in everyday use to explain some symptoms. Though not all of modern medicine is accepted, human experimentation is. There is some cultural resistance to human experimentation as well as to the idea of informed consent, and physicians and medical scientists oscillate between the values of modern medicine and those of traditional culture.

Resistance to human experimentation

"Physicians have been experimenting on their patients since time immemorial" (Schafer, 1982), or experimenting on themselves; according to a Chinese legend the Father of Chinese medicine (also the Father of Chinese agriculture), Shennong, "tasted a hundred species of herbs and exposed himself to seventy kinds of poison a day" (Liu), or "Medicine originated with Shennong who tasted a hundred species of herbs" (Sima). However, traditional Chinese medical texts have no word for 'experiment'. The word *shiyan*, which is the translation of the English 'experiment' or 'experimentation' in modern Chinese, was coined later. Practitioners of traditional Chinese

---

* Director, Programs in Bioethics, Institute of Philosophy, Chinese Academy of Social Sciences, Beijing, People's Republic of China.

medicine (TCM) never performed human experiments in the modern sense in its 2000-year history.

Two factors in Chinese culture, one epistemological, the other ethical, may explain why human experimentation was never invented in TCM, and why the Chinese public still resist, or are reluctant to accept, it.

All three main schools of philosophy, namely Confucianism, Taoism and Buddhism, developed an internalist approach, or "seeking the truth from within" — the concept that knowledge is gained from introspection rather than by observation.

One of the founders of Confucianism, Mencius, first advanced the concepts of innate ability, which is acquired without learning, and innate knowledge, which is possessed without deliberation, and the thesis that 'All is complete in me' (Chan 1963, pp. 80, 82). Another Confucian classic, *The Great Learning*, describes a comprehensive Confucian educational, moral and political programme, including the very influential 'eight steps': the investigation of things (*gewu*), the extension of knowledge, sincerity of the will, rectification of the mind, cultivation of the personal life, regulation of the family, national order, and world peace (Chan, pp. 84-94). Although later the imported 'physics' was translated into 'the learning of gewu', no science based on observation and experiment ever developed from *gewu* (investigation of things). In the later period Neo-Confucianists argued about the meaning of *gewu*. The proponents of the school of *li* (principle, the reason of being) argued that *li* is inherent in things, but that *li* had to be discovered by intuition during observation. The proponents of the school of *xin* (mind) argued that *li* is inherent in the mind, but it concealed wrong ideas — that is, non-sincerity — and *li* will be manifest only after correcting the wrong ideas (Chan, pp. 588-691).

Taoists developed a similar internalist approach. In the work of Guan Zi there is a chapter on internal endeavour, in which the author wrote:

"All things in the universe including grains, stars, spirits and gods, and sages are the product of *qi* (vital energy, air). *Tao*, life, thinking and knowledge, all presuppose the existence of *qi*. Keeping *qi* in the body, the person will get *Tao*, on which depends life or death, success or failure, and which sharpens his organs, clears his thinking, protects him from disease, and keeps his body intact. (How to keep *qi* in the body?) Controlling the mind. Controlling the mind is to keep it in calmness or stability. The mind is stable, you will be able to see and hear clearly, your limbs strong, *qi* in your body. If *qi* prevails, the world will be convinced; if the mind is stable, the world will listen to you."

The proponents of the most popular school of Buddhism in China — the Zen school — argued that the Buddha-nature is in all men, so that all can become Buddha. One of the Great Masters, Huineng, taught:

"Perfect wisdom is inherent in all people. It is only because they are deluded in their minds that they cannot attain enlightenment by themselves... Calmness and wisdom are foundations of my method. They are one substance and not two. Calmness is the substance of wisdom and wisdom is the function of calmness" (Chan, p. 433).

This internalist approach to the theory of knowledge has had great influence upon traditional Chinese science and medicine. Even as late as the 18th century the naturalist, Liu Xianting, wrote:

"It was said that a piece of iron could prevent a magnet from attracting another piece of iron and a test was performed to confirm this. (But) a test is unnecessary because it is only a trivial truth. It was also said that garlic could prevent a magnet from attracting a piece of iron as well. (But) I did not test it". (Jin *et al.*)

The practitioners of TCM also emphasized the internalist approach; for instance, an anonymous writer wrote:

"The *Tao* of practising medicine is that you must rectify yourself before you rectify things. To rectify yourself means to understand principles in order to bring your skill into full play. To rectify things means to treat patients with medication... If you have not rectified yourself, how can you rectify things? If you cannot rectify things, how can you cure a patient's disease?"

Even today practitioners of TCM maintain that experimentation on either human beings or animals is unnecessary. However, more and more, open-minded young TCM practitioners recognize the importance of experimentation.

The second factor incompatible with human experimentation is the ethical factor. The most popular Confucian ethical principle among the Chinese public, especially the traditionalists, is filial piety. According to this principle: "Hair and skin, which are imparted by parents, must not be damaged. This is the beginning of filial piety." (*The Book of Filial Piety*.)

However, 'hair and skin' may be damaged for parents' well-being. In traditional China there are 24 popular models of behaviour of the dutiful son, from various periods of history. One model is of a son whose ill parents wanted to have dinner with meat but were too poor to buy it, so the son cut a piece of flesh off his leg to feed his parents. The reasoning is simple: what parents impart they may permit it to be given back, but others may not.

On top of this cultural background there has been a more serious, politico-ideological, factor. In the 1950s when there was a widespread movement in China against American imperialism it became known

190

that American and Chinese doctors in the Peking Union Medical College had experimented on patients, without benefit to the patients, during the 1930s and 1940s. One example was the injection of cardiazol into an epileptic patient to observe its effect in inducing the seizure of epilepsy. The test had been filmed and when the film was shown during the anti-American movement it caused a sensation; the audience flew into a rage. Today, the audience and their children have forgotten 'American imperialism' but the after-effect continues: human experimentation is identified with the use of patients or subjects as guinea-pigs. Since that time many officials in the health administration and the public have been hostile to human experimentation.

Justification for human experimentation

I agree with the views of Englehardt (1986):

"Research is integral to medicine as to science" (p. 290).

"One need not only fear the reckless use of humans in medical research. One should also fear the costs of reckless treatment — treatment not based on adequate research" (p. 291).

"Research is integral to a beneficent medicine... One finds here yet one more application of the Socratic adage that the unexamined life is not worth living, namely, that medicine unexamined through systematic research may be a danger to patients" (p. 292).

The results of precluding human experimentation for a long period are serious. Underdeveloped or inefficacious therapies were widely used, some without being tested on humans. In the early 1950s, in a movement called 'Learning from the Soviet Union', Felatov's tissue was used throughout the country; some doctors even used it to treat pneumonia, with fatal results. During the Cultural Revolution officials of the Ministry of Health called for health workers to spread the therapy, as though it could cure all diseases. Also, in promoting acupuncture anaesthesia, they demanded its use in 90% of operations. This led to negative consequences, including the death of patients. Acupuncture can suppress pain and is a useful auxiliary to drug anaesthesia, but cannot replace it. After the Cultural Revolution the Ministry of Health no longer advocated the spread of some favoured therapy, but the public followed recurring fashions in therapy, such as chicken-blood therapy, swing arms therapy, red-tea fungus therapy, and *qigong* (deep breathing exercise) therapy, which spread one after another. These so-called therapies turned out to be useless or even harmful, and then were rejected one after another. Of course, we should not neglect some valuable folk therapies which people discovered by trial and error for treating illnesses that doctors could not cure or in which they were not interested. However, if they are to become optional therapies in medicine, they must be tested on animals and humans by scientific methods.

Secondly, a few medical researchers tested herbs or new drugs on themselves. Following Shennong's example, some bare-foot doctors tested herbs without precautions and died of poisoning.

Thirdly, the pharmaceutical industry in China manufactures many kinds of new drugs every year, many of which are used in clinics without human experimentation and widely advertised in newspapers. The advertisements cite favourable responses of patients and physicians, intended to persuade other physicians to use the drugs. Also, some foreign drug-companies have experimented with drugs on human subjects without informed consent and sometimes harmed patients.

Moreover, the rejection by TCM practitioners of experimentation had a fatal effect on traditional medicine. The prescientific test may distinguish betwen poisons and herbs, but can not distinguish between the effective and the ineffective substances in a herb, or quantify and standardize them. For instance, some practitioners prescribe one or two centipedes as an ingredient of a mixture, but others may use one hundred. Because there was no way to distinguish efficacious from non-efficacious substances in traditional therapies, some therapies were lost in competition. However, today, many TCM institutes carry out animal and human experiments.

Chinese experience has shown that a society cannot afford the costs of reckless and untested treatments. The principle of beneficence requires professionals to use tested medicaments and society to regulate untested medicaments.

Can human experimentation be ethically justified in the framework of Chinese culture? Chinese culture is sufficiently flexible to assimilate alien values and make them its own. The strategy might be as follows:

The rule of non-damage of the physical body must be rejected. It is a primary obligation from which exemption may be obtained if a conflicting obligation is given priority over it. The example cited above shows that the well-being of parents is more important than damage to the body. At the least, human experimentation is ethically permissible on the principle of filial peity, because it will result in a tested treatment, which will eventually benefit the subjects' parents.

Reinterpretation of filial piety

The principle of filial piety may be reinterpreted in accordance with the cardinal ethical principle of humaneness — 'loving others' (Confucius). Since participation as a subject in human experimentation will benefit society and mankind, it is ethically desirable according to the principle of humaneness.

Certain values in Chinese culture favour human experimentation. Confucianists emphasize the principles of solidarity and altruism. They argue that the only difference between human beings and animals is that human beings take others into account, but animals only themselves. Confucian ethics teaches people how to be human, on the basis of the principles of humanitarianism, solidarity and altruism. It promotes science and medicine as a collective endeavour.

Is human experimentation a moral obligation (Eisenberg) or a noble choice (Jonas)? It depends upon the belief or value system in which the judgement is made. If what is done will improve the condition of the world, according to a certain belief or value system, the action is obligatory; if it makes it worse, the action is prohibited; if the effect is uncertain, the action is permissible. But an action that is obligatory according to one belief or value system may be only permissible or even prohibited in another system. For example, Jonas argues that all non-therapeutic research involving human subjects infringes the individual's 'primacy inviolability'; in Kantian terms he objects to the use of a person as a means rather than an end. What is an end may depend upon the belief or value system. If an individual establishes the end to benefit people or make a contribution to society, then it cannot be said that in participating in an experiment as a subject he is being used as a means. Also, I do not agree with Jonas' view that progress, including medical progress, is an optional goal, not an unconditional commitment. Perhaps I come from a Third World country, but I think even in developed countries it is not only optional.

In China the ethical distinction must be made between legitimate human experimentation and the use of a subject as a guinea-pig, and the public must be told that the distinction is crucial for China. In the latter case the subject is made a passive object, merely to be acted upon (Jonas), but this is not the case when the requirement of informed consent is met.

Difficulties with informed consent

There are difficulties both in communicating and in receiving informed consent. Their causes are mainly cultural. In a country like China, where 25% of the population is illiterate or semi-literate, it is difficult to communicate effectively and exchange information, and to conduct a dialogue between a physician-researcher with advanced, sophisticated scientific knowledge and a patient-subject who is illiterate, from a remote rural area. This is clash of two cultures. The patient-subject entering the laboratory encounters a totally strange world, hearing an incomprehensible foreign language. The gap between experimenter and subject is so wide that researchers feel puzzled and depressed, but the gap is not unbridgable. Perhaps Chinese physician-researchers have not paid attention to developing the skills of conveying information about procedures, risks, alternatives and consequences to patient-subjects, and of helping them comprehend the information, making them sufficiently informed to be able to make valid decisions. The difficulty associated with informed consent may be due to a deeper element in the culture — its collective-oriented, holistic, socio-political philosophy.

Informed consent is based on the principles of beneficence and autonomy. The principle of autonomy requires that the individual's right of self-determination be respected. In cities or other advanced areas of China, educated people, more and more, have developed what I call the awakening of consciousness of their rights — that is, they claim the right to make their own individual decisions by themselves on issues that concern them.

However, this rights-oriented and individualistic approach is still under-developed. Since antiquity China has fostered the patriarchal clan system, which accorded the family's interests priority over the individual's interest, and then the family was taken as a model of the country. The king or emperor was no more than a patriarch of a big family. Confucianism and, later, Marxism further strengthened the collective-oriented and duty-oriented, holistic, socio-political philo-sphy. The patriarchal clan system is no more, but the family tie is still so strong that many decisions involving a family member are made by the family and not by the individual. In a clinic, decisions have usually been made on the basis of consultation between a patient's family and the physician, sometimes involving the patient's friends or colleagues or responsible fellow workers, but the final decision-maker is the patient's family, including the patient but not as an individual decision-maker. Sometimes the patient refuses to be informed or waives the right of self-determination. In the United States in the hospital of the National Institutes of Health, an American woman patient of Chinese origin refused to be informed and give consent, preferring her husband to act as her proxy. This embarrassed the physician. A colleague in the Bioethics Group consulted me about the case and I explained the position and suggested that her will be respected.

Response of physician-researchers to resistance
to human experimentation and difficulties with informed consent

Case 1

A herb (*Artemisia anna L.*) was recorded in Chinese medical texts as being an effective antipyretic, detoxicant and anti-malarial, and was also used as an anti-malarial in some parts of China. In 1972 an effective anti-malarial ingredient was isolated from the herb, with the molecular formula $C_{15}H_{22}O_5$. It was found to have such qualities as low toxicity, rapid absorption, wide distribution, and rapid excretion in experimental animals (cats, dogs, guinea-pigs, rabbits, rats and mice), and the ability to kill chloroquine-resistant plasmodia. Between 1973 and 1978 it was used in clinics to treat 2,099 malaria patients, with good effect, but the rate of short-term recurrence was relatively

194

high. To solve the problem, pharmacokinetic research on human subjects was designed. The conditions for participation included: healthy volunteers, voluntary consent, monitoring of subjects by physicians during the experiment, and the provision of subsidies for nutritional purposes to subjects after the experiment. Because of difficulty in enrolling volunteers the researcher made himself the first subject; the other three were also employees in the institute of pharmacology. The experiment was very successful. (Jin *et al.*). This is a typical case. Many volunteers are workers in institutes or hospitals and their families.

Case 2

To find an effective, non-toxic, and inexpensive drug to lower the blood-lipid level and morbidity and mortality from atherosclerosis, an experiment was performed on human subjects to determine whether oats could be used as a new medicine. A 73-year-old male patient with coronary and high-blood-lipid disease was assigned to the control group. In case he might be reluctant to participate in the research the researcher withheld some information: the patient was not told that he could be assigned to the control group. Later the patient noticed the difference between the drug being tested and the placebo, but still complied with the prescription (Jin *et al.*). The deliberate non-disclosure of pertinent information to the patient-subject violated the principle of autonomy.

Case 3

This is a 10-year cooperative project on the prevention of neural-tube defects, to be carried out by a Chinese institute and an American counterpart. Two countries have been selected as test fields. The project is still at the pre-test stage. The purpose of the experiment is to observe the effects of different doses of folic acid, and of different combinations of folic acid with multiple vitamins, upon the occurrence of neural-tube defects. It has been confirmed that folic acid is effective and has no known hazards for pregnant women or fetuses. Most of the prospective subjects (married or pregnant women) and their husbands had graduated from junior middle-school. The researcher showed them a videotape containing information on procedures, risks and consequences. However, the word 'experiment' or 'research' was not mentioned; instead was used the phrase 'observation of medicine's effect'. It was emphasized that participation would not only benefit the subjects, their families and future generations, but also contribute to the good of society and the world, because in China subjects cannot be enrolled for their own benefit only. Nevertheless, during the experiment subjects will have access to much better health care than others. They were also assured that there would be no discrimination

195

against anybody who refused to participate, or who withdrew at any time, or who would resume participation after withdrawal. After the videotape show the prospective subjects went home to discuss the matter with their families, and then gave their consent orally to the village doctor. So far, only three have declined to participate. Then the the village doctor signed the consent form as the representative of the community. The practice is called community consent. The project was approved by the institutional review bodies in both countries.

These cases are very illustrative of human experimentation and informed consent in China. Informed consent is a universal principle and should be applied in all countries. As Engelhardt (1986, p. 297) put it:

"To recognize individuals as free and able to consent or refuse to participate in research is to see science as the collective endeavor of a great number of free men and women. Those who govern its course are not only scientists, physicians, surgeons, and nurses, but patients and research subjects as well. ...when patients and others freely participate in research, they join in the collective endeavor of individuals concerned to avoid treatments that do more harm than good, to acquire treatments that cure better and with fewer costs, as well as in the general cultural aspiration to the better understanding of man and the human condition."

Deliberate non-disclosure of relevant information or deceiving a subject is morally wrong, violating the principles of beneficence and autonomy. In view of China's cultural diversity, the way in which informed consent is obtained may be adapted to the cultural context. In Chinese rural areas individual consent is inadequate for participation in human experimentation. If the heads of communities or families do not give consent, it will be difficult to obtain consent from individual villagers. However, the family or community has no right to decide which of its members should participate, and may not force anyone to give consent. Consequently, I prefer the term *informed consent with the aid of family or community* to the term *community consent*.

References

Chinese

Anon: *On Prescriptions of Pediatrics*.
Guan Zi, chapter Internal Endeavour.
Jin, D.J. *et al*: 1986, *Ethical Issues in Human Experimentation: Case Analysis*, presented at the Beijing Colloquium on Medical Ethics, unpublished.
Jin GT et al. (eds.): 1983, *Scientific Tradition and Culture*, Xian: Shaanxi Science & Technology Press.
Liu, An: *Huainan Zi*.
Qiu, R.Z.: 1987, The Development of Science-Technology and the Dilemmas Facing Chinese Medicine, *Studies in Dialectics of Nature* No. 3, 37-46.
Sima, Qian: *Records of the Historian*.

English and Spanish

Beauchamp, T.: 1989, Informed Consent, in: R. Veatch (ed.), *Medical Ethics*. Boston: Jones & Bartlett, pp. 173-200.

Capron, A.: 1989, *Human Experimentation, op. cit.*, pp. 125-172.

Chan, W.T.: 1963, *A Source Book in Chinese Philosophy*, Princeton, New Jersey: Princeton University Press.

Eisenberg, L.: 1977, The Social Imperatives of Medical Research, *Science* 198: 1105-1110.

Engelhardt, Jr., T.: 1986, *The Foundation of Bioethics*, New York, Oxford University Press, pp. 262-291.

Jones, H.: 1969, Philosophical Reflections on Experimenting with Human Subjects, *Daedalus* 98: 219-247.

Katz, J.: 1984, *The Silent World of Doctor and Patient*, New York, Free Press.

Qiu, R.Z.: 1987, Sobre la Tensión entre Internalismo y Externalismo en la Historia de la Ciencia, in: A Lafuente & J. Saldna (eds.), *Neuvas Tendencia: Historia de las Ciencias*. Madrid, Consejo Superior de Investigaciones Cientificas, pp. 25-39.

Schafer, A.: 1982, The Ethics of Randomized Clinical Trials, *New England Journal of Medicine*, 16: 719-724.

AN EASTERN MEDITERRANEAN PERSPECTIVE: ISLAMIC AND CULTURAL INFLUENCES

K.Z. Hasan*

As a prelude to this conference The Aga Khan University Medical College in Karachi, the Baqai Foundation, and the Department of Philosophy of Karachi University held a meeting, on the topic of this paper, of a group that included jurists, psychologists, religious scholars, medical scientists, sociologists and other concerned individuals. The meeting used the set of questions that form the agenda of this conference as the basis of discussion.

The first problem that the group identified was the wide gulf that exists in most Islamic, indeed all Third World, countries between the clerical and the professional groups. In traditional systems of medicine there was considerable interaction between the religious scholars and those who practised the healing arts. In the colonial era the traditional system was replaced by the Western system of medicine, which enjoyed the patronage of the colonial governments. The traditional systems were relegated to the background. The emerging and more dynamic Western systems were adopted particularly by the elites, who became more and more westernized. The two systems and their practitioners began to differ not only in content but also in form. In form, the economic levels, the modes of living and the social circles differed from the emerging Western-oriented, elite groups. The traditional practitioners continued to have more in common, and had more points of contact, with the religious and clerical groups than had the practitioners of modern systems of medicine. When the colonial era ended and was replaced by nationalist movements in many countries, attempts were made to bridge the gap that had developed in the colonial period. This process is exemplified in the subcontinent of India. The last of the Mogul kings was replaced by British rule in the early 19th century. During the Mogul period the system of medicine that had official sanction was called "Arabian Medicine". It was also called "Unani" or "Greek", which indicated its origin in the teaching of eminent Greek physicians, rendered accessible to the Muslim world. "It was in fact an eclectic synthesis of more ancient systems, chiefly Greek, but in a lesser degree Indian and old Persian, with a tincture of other exotic systems less easily to be identified..."[1]

The practitioners of that system were drawn from the same stratum of society as the clerical groups. Within an extended family system there were more points of intellectual contact and social intercourse. The gradual introduction of the modern medical system coincided with changes within society, and the process, inexorable as it was,

---

* Dean, Baqai Medical College, Karachi, Pakistan.

began to polarize society — the modern educated at one extreme and, at the other, the traditional medical groups along with the religious scholars.

In most developing countries medical ethics is not part of mainstream thought, not even in the medical profession. It is alluded to briefly whenever an instance of medical negligence or malpractice makes the headlines. The result is that discussion on ethical matters, which can become passionate in the West, is virtually absent in developing countries. One would expect that in a country where religious people also exercise political power such discussion would be fairly common and even intense, but even in Iran, which is one such country, medical ethics is not a major subject of discussion or concern. This is due to lack of mechanisms for establishing dialogue between representatives of different viewpoints. We have seen above how the systems of medicine became part of a sociopolitical process and how this led to increasing the distance between the systems.

Cultural perceptions in these countries are governed by prevailing religious thought. Also there is great diversity in Islamic thought. Islam has a very wide spread, from the eastern Atlantic coast to the western Pacific and from the temperate regions of the North to far South of the Equator. There are 1.2 billion Muslims, or 18.3% of the world's population, spread over 20% of the land-mass. Of these, 385 million live in the Eastern Mediterranean Region of the World Health Organization, constituting the vast majority of the population. Islam is embraced by peoples from a large number of ethnic and linguistic groups. Over the years these cultures have modified some of the basic principles of Islam to meet political and cultural exigencies. Islam's original message was to humanity as a whole. "Insan" or Man was the prime object. The main source of guidance is the Qur'an, followed by Hadith/Sunna, Ijmaa and Qiyas. Ijmaa is interpretation by people by consensus. Qiyas is analogy, which uses precedent as a basis for decisions. Ijtehad, which certain schools accept and others deny, depends on reasoning from basic principles for application to the immediate situation. Then comes the Aalim (the lawgiver). All of these are cultural adaptations with their roots in local circumstances.

Ethical values are universal but are deeply embedded in cultural contexts, as will be seen later. Their interpretation is also determined by the resources available to individuals, families and communities. Also, they are influenced heavily by prevailing economic and political systems. Over the years there has been much local interpretation, sometimes determined by political necessity but often by the social need to adapt to technological advance and cultural change. There are instances of original concepts being superseded for pragmatic reasons. Some interpretations appear to distort original concepts; others represent adaptation that remains true to the meaning but results in distortion in its application.

In theory at least, Islam gives considerable scope for personal autonomy. Islam recognizes many Prophets of God and their injunctions, which implies that it accepts that laws have to evolve to suit the needs of society as it changes. The teaching of the Qur'an is that life is a process of progressive creation, which requires that each generation, guided but unhampered by the work of its predecessors, should be permitted to solve its own problems. This is the way in which Allama Iqbal wanted to solve the predicament faced by the Ummah.

Islam believes that the finality is not in the immutability of legislation but rather in that there will be no more divine revelation, and that the legal system is left to be determined by the people according to their lights. This concept is specially applicable to individual autonomy. Paternalism was originally an integral part of tribal culture, in which decisions were taken collectively. As tribal societies evolved into feudal societies, collective decisions became family decisions. Family decision-making meets the needs of feudal societies, where paternalism on the part of the head of the family is both a protective mechanism and a significant factor in maintaining the economic system. In the West the evolution from paternalism to individual autonomy progressed at different rates in different cultures. In the United States and the Scandinavian countries individual autonomy was easily achieved. In France, Germany and the Soviet Union the process was accelerated by revolutionary changes that overthrew the feudal order. The movement towards individual autonomy has been slower in the United Kingdom and Japan. Islamic countries are part of the Third World, where these social and political changes have not taken place, and progress towards political autonomy has been extremely slow. Society in developing countries is essentially traditional and focuses on the family rather than the individual. This has influenced all aspects of life. Paternalism is a mode of life, exercised within the family. The family wants the physician to exercise paternalism. Withholding the truth is not lying. It is believed that truth can sometimes be harmful to some people if they are not "spiritually" strong. The practice ranges from giving all the information (which may not be absorbed or accepted or properly handled), to censoring (withholding some information), to fabrication and deception. Islam prohibits deception but allows "withholding truth if it creates mischief". Major transitions in social life have also been affected by growth in science and technology. Culture is a reflection of not only religious trends in a society but also political and economic trends.

Reference

1. Browne, E.G. 1921, *Arabian Medicine*. Cambridge University Press.

A LATIN AMERICAN PERSPECTIVE

G. Soberón*, M. Tarasco**, J. Kuthy**

It has been stated that human values are the basis of the ethics of research involving human beings and, in a more general way, of the ethics of the professional practice of medicine. Human values are manifested and expressed in different ways and with different sensitivities in different cultural settings, and consequently the same is true of ethical judgements. Our paper is based on our experience in Mexico and its possible extrapolation to the other Latin American countries with which we have basic links such as language, religion and historical experience — in short, ways of being, thinking and acting.

Some special characteristics of Latin American countries with regard to research involving human subjects

The culture that shapes the idiosyncrasy of human beings will influence the way in which research is carried out. Moreover, this same culture may be that of the researcher, thus leaving its characteristic seal on each side of the research coin.

Some of these culturally determined characteristics will be expressed as variants of research in humans.

The Catholic religion is predominant in Latin America, although today new and very different religions are proliferating in the continent and will have a political and economic influence on the population. At the same time, the indigenous legacy is expressed in a strong sense of magic, and a fatalist way of thinking. Nevertheless, the Catholic religion, which promotes ethical and moral principles that support man's dignity, determines some of the characteristics of the continent's large and heterogenous population.

The family structure is strong, despite the high incidence of disintegrated family nuclei, which is due to paternal absence, especially among the underprivileged social sectors. The extended family, which comprises not only parents and offspring but also grandparents, uncles, cousins, and even the children of a mistress, compensates for a missing parent and supports a whole structure of standards and traditions that result in close relationships in which the obligations and rights of each family member are recognized and respected.

This situation benefits the elderly, for they are cared for by family members with a greater solidarity than is found in other countries, sometimes providing even economic support to family members in need. Such close family ties create complex social relations, which, to some extent even at high socio-economic levels and in large cities, influence community decisions.

---

* Mexican Health Foundation, Mexico City, Mexico.
** Bioethics Department, Universidad Anahuac, Mexico City, Mexico.

The low average level of education fosters a dependency on, and fear of, those that represent authority, granting them a magic value because of their capacity or ability to resolve problems. This also makes the population more vulnerable to being used for unethical experiments or at least for non-useful procedures, which with the underlying fatalistic attitude of the people fosters an irresponsibity that can lead to the failure of any research work.

The endemic diseases of Latin American countries depend not only on geographical and climatological factors, but also on the low average level of education, which contributes to the perpetuation of low standards of hygiene and to lack of interest in increasing knowledge on medical and health topics.

There is the fact also that our clinical research is little known abroad, for our national journals are frequently not indexed in *Index Medicus*. Consequently, our authors do not receive the credit they deserve and valuable material is wasted which could be reported in other publications with a broad scientific readership.

There is a considerable amount of clinical research in Latin America. The meetings of the different medical specialties are saturated by reports of work carried out in institutional and private hospitals. A large part is of sufficiently high quality to stimulate discussion and encourage scientific research in our own countries but is not published in journals recognized internationally.

In Mexico, the National Council for Science and Technology has reported that 60% of research is clinical, 30% basic biomedical, and 10% public health. Obviously there is an urgent need to increase research in public health, to provide much needed epidemiological and health systems information.

Not all health institutions can undertake clinical research. Adequate research is not possible where the pressure of health-care demands leaves the researcher no time to prepare sound protocols. Institutional structures should permit a research hierarchy to complement health care and teaching.

Some basic issues in research involving humans:
principles, procedures, standards

In considering the ethical aspects of experimentation with human beings, it should be understood that such experimentation includes not only research in its usual sense but also the use of human beings for the training of medical students or other health-care professionals.

Experimentation with human beings is the basis of learning and is applied in medicine, as when medical students use for the first time techniques that previously they had studied only theoretically or had observed others using. Such experimentation requires ethical regulation to ensure adequate medical training and avoid risk to patients. Thus, research involving humans can have a pragmatic sense in that, after carrying out a series of actions, the "subject" acquires new knowledge.

In this respect ethical standards can be violated. It is common, for instance, in low-income areas, such as rural districts and health-care facilities of underprivileged areas on the outskirts of large cities, where medical students or poorly trained physicians use health-care techniques they have not mastered and do so without adequate supervision.

Another issue of concern to expert researchers is the decision whether to intervene in the disease process or to withhold intervention in favour of observation of the natural course of a disease or administering a placebo.

Intervention implies assessing risks to the subject; observation or the administration of a placebo may represent the denial of a benefit that might result from an intervention, apart from any psychological effect of the placebo. In any case, it is essential to respect the autonomy and the capacity of the subject, and to follow correct procedures for obtaining the consent of the individual. These issues have already been widely discussed and therefore need not be dwelt on here.

The experimental stages of human-subject research which are required to be carried out in animals are subject to ethical control, and, although this aspect of ethics is not addressed at this conference, it is of interest that public opinion is much less rigorous on this matter in Latin America than in other countries. However, in the assessment of the protocol the use of non-endangered species is required as well as the use of methods that avoid unnecessary pain in animals.

Since risk is a distinctive aspect of human experimentation, it is necessary to define who are the subjects of such experimentation: patients, health-sector volunteers, or subjects deprived of freedom of choice. The ethical consideration is to establish the values underlying experimentation and the conditions for ensuring minimal risk in its different phases and stages.

The major aim of analysing the ethical aspects of a project is to determine the primary purpose of the study and assess whether the basic ethical principles have been respected from the beginning of the scientific process and the integrity of the human being is fully respected.

Serrano-LaVertu and Linares point out three basic ethical principles: respect for individuals, the benefit of the individuals, and a fair selection for risks and benefits. Also, they explain why experimentation in humans has been carried out in developing countries, generally by researchers of developed countries. Among the reasons they give are: the prevalence of uniquely regional diseases, which obviously can be studied only in the endemic populations; the lower costs of research in developing countries than in industrialized countries; and insufficient legislation on this matter in Third World countries, which permits researchers to omit in these countries requirements imposed in other countries.

An additional aspect should be pointed out: the populations that "suffer" experimentation should also be able to receive its benefits, and it is precisely these populations that, in a large number of cases, do not receive the benefits, because of the cost of the new scientific product.

The discussion on human rights and biomedical progress is taking place in an historic context that offers new possibilities and responsibilities, because the ethical question has been defined.

Elio Sgreccia considers four facts that result from a lack of ethical standards and that over time have been responsible for gross violations of the integrity of individuals:

1. *A greater awareness of the limits of science in the philosophical field and therefore the predominance of a pragmatic viewpoint derived from the potential of experimental science, especially in relation to medical science.*

   In this respect philosophy states that experimental science is not the only way of knowing reality. Wittgenstein, an analyst philosopher, has written: "If all possible questions of science could be answered, we would only be starting to deal with the problems of our life."

   Another reaction to scientism has come from the philosophical trend of phenomenology: Scheller and Hertman demand a space for the only values that can give sense to human life.

   Existentialists say that scientific knowledge cannot offer any direction to humans, since it cannot establish valid values.

2. *Scientific and technological progress in biology and medicine has raised the problem of the limit of human-subject research, in the interests of safeguarding the human being.*

   The progress of medicine has given great relevance to its biological basis. This has arisen from a legitimate desire to increase the scope of medical therapeutic research. It has been emphasized that there is no point in curing a disease if its cause has not been investigated, but although this is a totally legitimate point of view there is an ethical limit: that research will not be diverted to the manipulation of human life, as would be the case in gene manipulation, with positive as well as negative possibilities.

3. *Insufficient standards in the medical field regarding the ethics of professional conduct.*

   The pronouncement of law as "mutant and relative" *vis-à-vis* absolute values implicitly confronts law and ethics.

   In Latin America, despite the creation of ethics committees in hospitals of different countries, the relationship between the committees have a weak legal basis and in most of the countries the public are unaware of mechanisms for asserting their legal rights.

In Mexico we have the General Health Act, but although it has brought about some improvements its application lags behind today's rapid technological changes.

4. *The growing centralization of research and health-care practice in powerful political and economic groups, which determine the selection of research programmes that influence human life conditions.*

In the past, Latin American scientists have not been able to systematically sensitize the public and the governments to the relevance to society of scientific research, although during the past ten years there has been some progress in respect of biomedical research, to which more resources are now being allocated.

The task of physicians, both clinicians and researchers, who wish to promote science to create an adequate labor market for researchers should be to convince institutions of the actual and potential benefits of clinical research in bringing about a greater understanding of the basic mechanisms of diseases affecting Latin American populations.

In this continent, all these factors interact and result in the existence of groups of persons who, though not concerned directly with research, are responsible for decisions in this field because they have the economic means to do so, as in the case of the pharmacological industry.

Growing interest in bioethics

Rapid progress in medical technology, and the associated increase in research involving human subjects, have highlighted the need for bioethical regulation of the research and a closer surveillance of risks. There is therefore a growing interest in bioethics and an awareness of the need to deal with complex ethical problems.

This is illustrated by the case of Mexico in recent years. In 1984 the General Health Act was promulgated, which gave effect to a constitutional amendment establishing the right of every citizen to health protection. The Act requires each hospital to create a research committee, an ethics committee, and a biosafety committee.

In 1987 the Regulation on Health Research was approved, which defines ethical standards to be strictly observed in research involving human beings, in relation to such matters as: the scientific basis of the research, previous research experience with laboratory animals or human beings, risk assessment, relevance of the knowledge sought, expected benefits, and the competence of the research groups.

The Bioethics Academy was created in 1987 to carry out studies and research, and to publicize developments, in bioethics.

In 1990 the School of Medicine, Universidad Anáhuac, created the Institute of Humanism in Medicine, which includes among its tasks the teaching of bioethics.

Since 1980 the National Academy of Medicine has collaborated with CIOMS in reviewing the exercises carried out in Mexico regarding the Proposed International Guidelines for Biomedical Research Involving Human Subjects.

Despite these developments interest in bioethics has been confined largely to medical care and health institutions, and still needs to be extended to other fields.

Some topics of bioethical interest

It is convenient to mention some illustrative examples of the aspects that have caused debate regarding the adequate operation of health-care workers, the subjects involved in experimentation, and the interested sector of society.

Family planning. In Mexico, in the early 1970s, annual population-growth rates reached 6.5%. In 1974 legislation was introduced and policies were established for controlling demographic growth, based mainly on family planning. Despite initial reservations about contraceptive methods and more permissive sexual practices, and some resistance on religious grounds, the effect has been to reduce the total fertility rate from 6.5 during the 70s to 3.3 at present, and a decrease in the population-growth rate to 2%.

Artificial insemination. Procedures for artificial insemination and "surrogate pregnancy" have been introduced, accompanied by expressions of concern about genetic manipulation and lack of respect for the dignity of individuals, but the discussion has been restricted to those more directly involved.

Abortion. Abortion is illegal in Mexico except when the mother's life is at risk and for pregnancy due to rape. However, more than 600,000 cases of abortion are treated annually, many of which are induced, but without any legal prosecutions. There are no reliable data on morbidity and mortality associated with abortion, although estimates indicate it is an important cause of maternal mortality and, therefore, a public health problem. Several attempts to legalize abortion have encountered violent reaction, mainly political, from pressure groups with religious affiliations. Recently, a bill passed by the government of Chiapas to legalize abortion was cancelled as a result of the opposition it generated.

Organ donations for transplant. There is growing acceptance of the donation of organs for transplant and there are new laws to specify the conditions for certifying that death has occurred and for the use of organs. With regard to embryonic tissue transplant, it has been necessary to define criteria, since the procedure is being used for some neuropathies. The Ministry of Health requested the Institute of Neurology and Neurosurgery to draw up a definition, and a group created expressly for this purpose declared the following:

"the embryo, from its conception, should be considered as an individual in all respects; that death, and not brain death, should be certified; that in the case of an embryo (less than 12 weeks of gestation), no death certification is required and, therefore, it can be used for transplants, with the consent of parents and the due protection of the recipient; that fetuses require death certification from physicians other than those involved in the transplant; and that in all cases it should be certified that the tissue is in an adequate biological condition to be considered as useful tissue for such purpose."

Health brigades. In recent years groups of physicians and medical students of foreign universities have formed groups that perform certain surgical procedures. In most cases, these interventions represent the altruistic aim of supporting low-income populations, but in others the intention of "using practice material" is clear. The objectives are often not clearly specified and the informed consent of the populations involved is not obtained. Neither is there adequate follow-up of surgical patients nor the least intention to assess results. Such activities are frequently carried out without the knowledge of health authorities; for this reason they are called "health safaris". Now, we are proposing that these activities be properly organized and regulated.

AIDS. The AIDS pandemic has resulted in ethical problems shared by all affected countries, mainly in regard to confidentiality of diagnostic procedures and discrimination against patients and seropositive individuals.

Education campaigns have met opposition in certain sectors, especially regarding the use of condoms. This opposition went to the extreme of accusing one of us (GS) before the Attorney General of being a corruptor of minors, for his responsibility in the organization of educational campaigns in his position as Minister of Health. However, a more straightforward vocabulary is now accepted and these objectives have been overcome.

The definition of standards and their frequent updating, the serious debate, the responsible participation of the citizen, and especially of health workers, and the study of procedures followed in other countries will lead us to make headway in combining technology with ethics. This is an essential service that society owes to itself.

A NORTH AMERICAN PERSPECTIVE

Charles R. McCarthy*

Before I comment on the specific task at hand, I should like to express my gratitude and appreciation to the staff of CIOMS and WHO, whose hard work and warm hospitality have made this such a successful conference. I should also like to express my gratitude to the participants in the conference from all parts of the world, who, despite their diverse cultural backgrounds and experience, have outlined a policy that expresses remarkable unity.

In particular I should like to recognize the work of Dr Zbigniew Bankowski, Secretary General of CIOMS. Few individuals of our time have made contributions that can equal that of our host and leader, Dr Bankowski. He recognized many years ago that, if we were to find ways to improve the health and well-being of the poor and the marginalized members of the world community, there must be developed cross-cultural understanding and deep respect for the traditions and the values of all peoples throughout the world. He also recognized that in a fundamental sense the principles that govern ethical research and ethical health care delivery must apply worldwide. His deep respect for values and traditions of the Third World, and his intuitive recognition that underlying principles can be applied in ways that promote unity while respecting cultural diversity, have been an inspiration. It would be ungracious of us to leave this meeting without recognizing the remarkable and lasting contribution that he has made.

Let us turn our attention to the work in hand, namely, providing guidance and insight to those who will redraft and update the 1983 CIOMS Guidelines for the Protection of Human Research Subjects. I have deliberately left the word "provisional" out of the title of those Guidelines because it has proved to be misleading and should not be included in the title of the new guidelines.

We have heard in the course of this meeting considerable discussion concerning two major points: (1) whether the principles of respect for persons, beneficence and justice can or should be incorporated into the new guidelines; and (2) whether the standards of conduct endorsed by the developed nations of the world can be applied to developing nations.

I should like to address each of these issues in turn.

Let us consider the three principles (respect for persons, beneficence and justice) set forth in the Belmont Report, issued by the U.S. National Commission for the Protection of Human Subjects of Biomedical and Behavioral Research, in 1978.

---

* Former Director, Office for Protection from Research Risks, National Institutes of Health, Bethesda, MD 20892, U.S.A.

On the one hand, we have heard eloquent arguments for incorporating these principles into the new guidelines. The arguments in support of including the principles may be summarized as follows: The principles are adumbrated in such illustrious sources as the Nuremberg Code and the Universal Declaration of Human Rights. They have proved remarkably effective in providing guidance to biomedical-research investigators throughout the United States, Canada, Australia and the United Kingdom. They have been subscribed to by institutions in more than 80 countries, across a wide cultural spectrum. They are gradually coming to be internalized by both investigators and research subjects throughout the Western World and in Asia, Africa and South America. In short, they have been applied by most of the countries in which biomedical research is conducted, and they have become a part of the culture of a number of the countries that conduct the largest portion of biomedical research in the world. The principles are broad enough to encompass the most diverse cultures, and flexible enough to allow for reasonable application in diverse cultures and in difficult cases.

On the other hand, we have heard these same principles derided as being little more than a "Georgetown [University] Mantra", which places principles in rigid hierarchy. Cases have been cited in which the principles have been applied in a way that distorts sound ethical values and distracts attention from the Helsinki Declaration, which has been periodically updated and which provides a superior framework for the conduct of research involving human subjects.

How can we reconcile these two positions?

My personal view is that the principles of respect for persons, beneficence and justice are time-tested and necessary, but not sufficient for the new CIOMS guidelines. They are necessary because it is inconceivable that research involving human subjects can be conducted without recognizing the dignity of the human subjects, without determining that the risks to research subjects are reasonable in the light of expected benefits to the subjects or to society as a whole, and without providing an equitable distribution of both the burdens and the benefits of research. To fail to meet any of these standards in research is to fail to conduct the research in an ethical manner.

Nevertheless, the CIOMS guidelines are to be applied throughout the world and particularly throughout the Third World. In this context, there is little doubt that the primary ethical concern must be to create a moral context in which the research will be pursued. That context must meet, at the very least, fundamental standards of justice. It is justice that has been stressed above all else by the delegates to this conference. Without justice, the other two principles are vacuous. It makes little sense to respect the dignity of individual subjects so long as the research is ongoing, but to simultaneously neglect the inequities in the community in which the subjects live. On the contrary, justice requires that Third World partners receive a reasonable share of the fruits of research. Further, justice demands that investigators from developed nations distribute the burdens and benefits of research equitably.

I would therefore hope that justice will be given the first place in the new guidelines, but that it will be supported by the other two principles. I can see no objection to referencing the Helsinki Declaration as well. The Helsinki document provides a level of detail and examples of application of the principles of justice, beneficence, and respect for persons. Surely it is too narrow a view to suggest that the principles are not in harmony with the Declaration. Both should be stressed.

I would add one more point. It is this: The principles have achieved notoriety in countries that stress individual liberty and place less emphasis on the rights and dignity of the community. However, many Third World communities have much to teach the developed nations about community values. For this reason I believe that the principles of justice, beneficence and respect for persons should be supplemented by a fourth principle, dealing with respect for the family and the community of the research subjects.

Turning to the second question, my comments can be very brief. I reject the notion that developed nations may conduct or support in foreign populations research that would not be acceptable in a domestic population. A double standard of morality would manifest hypocrisy on the part of the developed nations and unacceptable subservience on the part of the developing nations. Therefore it is imperative that the new guidelines express consistent standards that can meet the moral demands of all nations. To demand less would be to reject the principles of the Nuremberg Code; it would be to reject the Universal Declaration of Human Rights of the United Nations; and it would introduce unacceptable double standards of morality, demeaning to both developed and developing countries.

This is not to say that a certain cultural flexibility should not be allowed. Rigidity in application of common principles must be avoided. To demand that informed consent always be in writing, or never involve anyone other than the research subject, would be an example of unreasonable rigidity. But the guidelines should make it clear that abandoning informed consent because it is not well established in a given culture would be unacceptable to both those who conduct the research and those who are asked to participate.

I should like to emphasize this final point by citing a new provision in the regulations that now govern all research conducted or supported by the departments or agencies of the United States Government. What follows is a quotation from Sec. 101 (h) of the Code of Federal Regulations, Title 45, Part 46, issued on June 18, 1991.

When research covered by this policy takes place in foreign countries, procedures normally followed in the foreign countries to protect human subjects may differ from those set forth in this policy... In these circumstances, if a Department or Agency head determines that the procedures prescribed by the institution afford protections that are at least equivalent to those provided in this policy, the Department or Agency head may approve the substitution of the foreign procedures in lieu of the procedural requirements in this policy.

I submit to this body that it can take a giant step toward universal protection for human research subjects by drafting a new set of guidelines that can meet the "at least equivalent" standard of the U.S. regulations. To do less would set up a rivalry between U.S. regulations (the most widely used standards in the world) and the CIOMS guidelines (the second most widely used). To meet the challenge of "at least equivalent" would allow nations to choose CIOMS guidelines to meet U.S. funding requirements. Failure to meet the "at least equivalent" clause would almost certainly cause not only the U.S. but also institutions in 80 other nations to turn away from the guidelines.

We have a golden opportunity to achieve world harmony in support of common standards for the protection of human subjects. *Carpe diem!*

A EUROPEAN PERSPECTIVE

Sir Raymond Hoffenberg*

Every country that subscribes to a code of biomedical ethics now holds it necessary for all experimental protocols for research on humans to be submitted to specially-appointed independent ethics committees (ECs). Such committees exist in most European Community countries but it is doubtful whether sufficient conformity of opinion exists to constitute an agreed "European perspective". Reflecting on the comments made by Dr Levine, I would judge the European approach to be less pragmatic, more idealistic. Perhaps the memory of Nazi "experimentation" is still too close and vivid for the emphasis to fall anywhere but most strongly on the protection of the individual; the interests of science or the investigator are distinctly subservient to this. In Europe, too, we are less subject to pressure from (understandably) self-interested groups, e.g. those suffering from or at risk of AIDS or specific forms of cancer, and who demand that rigid scientific protocols should be waived in order to give them the chance to benefit from new, albeit scientifically-untested, drugs.

Most European countries have entrenched systems for promulgating ethical codes and for enforcing adherence to them. Indeed, most have — or are moving towards — a system of regional or local ethical committees with responsibility to approve and supervise the conduct of all research involving humans, carried out within their locality. A question arises about the legal status of such committees and the legal force of their judgements. The Committee of Ministers of the Council of Europe recommended in 1990 that member states should adopt legislation "or take any other measures" to ensure the implementation of their Stated Principles, No. 15 of which says "all proposed medical research plans should be the subject of an ethical examination by an independent and multidisciplinary committee". In France, Law No. 88-1138, which came into force on 31 December 1990, makes it obligatory for each Region to establish one or more Advisory Committees for the Protection of Participants in Biomedical Research, which "shall have legal personality". In the Netherlands a law will shortly be submitted to Parliament which will guarantee the rights of persons participating in research; submission of research protocols to a medical EC will be obligatory and its findings will "have the status of a binding recommendation"; a Central Committee will accredit ECs. In Italy there is no federal law but several regions have their own laws governing ECs. In Britain the Department of Health has recently stated that local research ethics committees must be responsible for considering all research projects that involve National Health Service patients, their records or the use of National Health

---

* President, Wolfson College, Oxford, England.

Service premises or facilities; they may advise on but have no jurisdiction over research not involving National Health Service patients, records or premises, e.g. in the private sector, Medical Research Council establishments or universities.

Even where the requirement to obtain EC approval for research is not legally enforceable, there is strong pressure to do so. In Britain, for instance, the Royal College of Physicians of London, which in 1967 advocated the universal establishment of local ECs, has issued guidelines for their practice (in 1984 and 1990); failure to comply with them would be viewed seriously by a court of law if, for instance, indemnity were being sought for damage incurred during experimentation. There are other strong sanctions: The Medical Research Council and other major charities will not fund research that has not received EC approval; employers can apply pressure; and editors may refuse to publish the results of work carried out without proper approval.

Within Europe there is broad general agreement about the constitution of local ECs and their method of practice. Assessment of the scientific validity of a project is thought to fall within the remit of an EC. The intention to involve humans — or animals, for that matter — in research that is scientifically dubious or unlikely to achieve acceptable results is in itself unethical. Where necessary, it is accepted that outside expert advice might be sought. There is less clarity about financial aspects. It is generally agreed that persons should not be subject to any inducement (financial or other) to participate. A contrary view has been expressed, especially by students and young unemployed people, that payment for voluntary participation in research projects is justified, that it can be seen as a job with far less exposure to risk than, say, work in the building trade, on oil-rigs or down a mine.

In the Council of Europe Recommendation No. R(90)3, the Revised Helsinki Declaration of 1989 and the current CIOMS draft, there is no consideration of the financial arrangements under which investigators undertake a study. Difficulties have arisen, especially in research sponsored by a pharmaceutical company, where payments to the investigators have been so large as to induce a few unscrupulous doctors to recruit patients improperly, e.g. by stopping perfectly satisfactory treatment in order to put them on a new drug under trial and, even, to "invent" non-existent participants to meet a contractual number of subjects. Such abuse is particularly liable to occur with payments made on a per capita basis, which the Royal College of Physicians of London believes may be unethical. Guiding Principle 4 of the CIOMS document states that all benefits intended to be provided to research subjects should be approved by an EC.

The Royal College of Physicians of London believes *all* aspects of payment — to investigators, participants or institutions — should be disclosed to and scrutinised by an EC. A particular problem might arise where volunteers participate in more than one project simultaneously, without informing the investigators; this may constitute a risk to their health as well as negating the outcome of the research. The opening-up of employment possibilities throughout Europe might tend to exacerbate the problem, and consideration should be given to the establishment of a computerized European register of all research participants, based on individual identification, e.g. by a passport, to avoid multiple enrolment.

The general principle that no medical research should be carried out without the "informed, free, express and specific consent" of the subject is widely accepted. There is a feeling that a signed consent form tends to be viewed as protection for investigators rather than subjects, and that the emphasis should be on providing information to the subjects' satisfaction and recording that this has been done. Figure 1 shows a proposed form for patient research, published by the Royal College of Physicians of London.

Figure 1. Proposed form for patient research

TITLE OF PROJECT
(The patient should complete the whole of this sheet himself/herself)   Please cross out as necessary
Have you read the Patient Information Sheet? ....   YES/NO
Have you had an opportunity to ask questions and discuss this study? ....   YES/NO
Have you received satisfactory answers to all of your questions? ....   YES/NO
Have you received enough information about the study? .....   YES/NO
Who have you spoken to? Dr/Mr/Ms ....
Do you understand that you are free to withdraw from the study:

• at any time,
    • without having to give a reason for withdrawing
    • and without affecting your future medical care? ....   YES/NO

Do you agree to take part in this study? ....   YES/NO
Signed .... **Date** ....
(NAME IN BLOCK LETTERS): ....

An important question concerns compensation for those who suffer injury as a result of participating in research. The Council of Europe accepts the need, and the CIOMS document states that the sponsor, whether a pharmaceutical manufacturer, a government or an institution, should agree before the research begins to pay compensation for any injury, obtaining insurance if necessary to cover compensation independent of proof of fault. In Britain the position is unsatisfactory; in law the right to compensation depends on a successful claim for negligence, but various bodies, such as the Medical Research Council and the Association of the British Pharmaceutical Industry, are able to make *ex gratia* payments. The National Health Service, which accepts responsibility for the ethical assessment of all human research carried out under its auspices, rejects any responsibility to offer advance indemnity to participants, and merely says that subjects of research, volunteers or patients, should be told at the outset what arrangements apply. Italy, France, Germany and the Netherlands all insist on adequate insurance cover being taken out by the sponsoring agency to indemnify participants without need for them to show negligence; to my knowledge, in Germany this applies only to pharmaceutical trials, not yet to all medical experimentation.

A final word about the accountability of ECs. Because of historical differences in the ways ECs have developed in different countries, there are divergent systems for ensuring their continued sound practice. In Italy, in which ECs appeared sporadically and independently, there appears to be no mechanism for auditing their performance. In Germany, appointing authorities such as medical councils and universities have some supervising functions, but all ECs meet once a year and have formed an umbrella organization. In France ECs are appointed by the Minister responsible for health in each Region, so presumably monitoring of their performance takes place through the Ministry. The proposed new law in the Netherlands will create a central committee for accrediting and supervising ECs. In the United Kingdom all ECs are now required to submit an annual report to the local health authority, which is open to public scrutiny; regular meetings of representatives of ECs are held under the auspices of the Royal College of Physicians of London.

Conclusion

This report is by no means comprehensive. I have selected a few topics from the multiplicity of aspects of biomedical research covered by the CIOMS and other documents and I have compared the treatment of these topics in the few European countries for which I have been able to get adequate information. It is clear that the general principles enunciated in the CIOMS document have been adopted by most if not all countries in Europe. The fact that there are divergences of approach simply reflects historical differences in the way in which awareness of these ethical issues has been translated into practice. As time passes, no doubt, differences will be eliminated and a unified and authoritative European code of bioethics will emerge.

References

Royal College of Physicians of London (1984) *Guidelines on the practice of Ethics Committees in medical research.* Report of the Royal College of Physicians of London.

Royal College of Physicians of London (1990) *Guidelines on the practice of Ethics Committees in medical research involving human subjects.* 2nd edition. Report of the Royal College of Physicians of London.

CONCLUSIONS AND IMPLICATIONS FOR ACTION

Robert J. Levine

As we take the next step in revising the Guidelines, the transcripts of the many fine presentations and discussions we have heard at this Conference will be highly influential. We will be especially attentive to the reports of the working groups; these well-developed and well-organized reports were distinctly responsive to the questions presented to them by the Steering Committee. Given the types of language barrier the working groups had to contend with, their accomplishments are quite remarkable. Their members came from many countries, with primary languages ranging from Arabic to Yoruba, to share their concerns in English. Even more formidable were the types of language barrier that were brought to our attention by Professors Solbakk, de Wachter, Gillon, and others — the language barriers presented by our unresolved conceptual and metaethical considerations.

In the next stage of development of the Guidelines we must concern ourselves with several issues that came up during this Conference.

First, let us consider the issue of providing payment or other material inducements to research subjects. During this Conference it became clear that the meaning of such inducements is very much related to the cultural context in which they are offered. Their meanings must be evaluated in the context of the gift-exchange traditions of the culture. It will be necessary to rely on research ethics committees with a thorough understanding of the cultural context to determine the propriety or lack of propriety of any material inducement that might be proposed.

Next, I wish to react to the suggestions that scientific review could be handled by a research ethics committee and that this committee should be located in the initiating country. Thorough scientific review is found problematic even by the most sophisticated research ethics committees in the most technologically advanced countries. The scientific review of plans to evaluate investigational new drugs, for example, requires toxicological expertise. Even in the United States there are not enough toxicologists to go around; there are many more research ethics committees than there are toxicologists. Similarly, thorough scientific review often requires expertise in such disciplines as pharmacology, immunology, microbiology, and statistics. For these and other reasons, it would be very difficult to develop local research ethics committees which have all of the expertise necessary to conduct thorough scientific review. However, it is generally unnecessary.

Most research proposals are funded by agencies of the government or by private philanthropic organizations; such agencies customarily provide very careful scientific review by a panel of experts in the field of study. Such reviews form the bases of their decisions about funding research proposals. Research ethics committees ordinarily need not repeat this review. For this reason, the standard for the research ethics committee should be to assure that thorough scientific review is accomplished by some competent agency, not necessarily or typically itself. In the case of research sponsored by a pharmaceutical company, responsibility for scientific review may be assigned to some other competent agency; scientific review committees may be established within drug registration agencies or medical research councils or within universities or other institutions in which the research is carried out.

The suggestion that scientific review in the initiating country might of itself be sufficient implies a belief that the standards for scientific design are universal. Even in science the standards are not quite as universal as they might seem to those who are not scientists. I am not at this point referring to the societies about which we heard this afternoon — those which do not even recognize the validity of our definition of research, the pursuit of generalizable knowledge, because it is believed that true knowledge is always individual and not generalizable.

I am now concerned with the fact that, in societies which define research as an activity designed to contribute to the development of generalizable knowledge, there are constantly trade-offs in scientific design according to the priorities of the society. Consider, for example, the design of a randomized clinical trial. A high level of confidence in the validity (accuracy) of the results is usually the dominant consideration in its design. Almost always, however, two other values compete with validity and with each other: generalizability (the results are widely applicable) and efficiency (the trial is affordable and resources are left over for patient care and other biomedical research). Generalizability can be increased by widening the criteria for inclusion of patients as subjects so that the results will be applicable, for example, to patients in all stages of the disease and to patients having various coexisting diseases. If this is not accompanied by an increase in the number of subjects, there will necessarily be a decrease in the validity of the results. Increasing numbers of subjects, of course, increases the expense of the study, thus reducing efficiency. The need to make decisions about such trade-offs is inescapable; sound judgments on such matters require expertise in the relevant sciences as well as familiarity with the values of the society in which the research is to be conducted.

The sanctions that have been recommended by the working groups for those who violate ethical standards in the conduct of research are directed primarily toward those who would commit these transgressions. Two of them, however, are likely to punish society as well as the wrong-doer. If we preclude publication of the results of research conducted unethically, then nobody will ever get the good of the knowledge that has been developed. There is a growing body of opinion that the results of research done unethically should be published accompanied by an editorial which calls attention to the appearance of ethical impropriety; in such cases the investigators should be invited to provide a response in which they defend their actions. Similarly, in the case of research designed to develop data to support applications for registration of drugs, devices or vaccines, it was proposed that we could forbid registration. But if a very good new therapy were developed, would we want to deprive society of its benefits? I think not. There are other devices available to sanction errant researchers without harming society's interests.

During this meeting we have had extensive discussion of whether and how the ethical principles should be presented in the revised Guidelines. Nearly all conferees support inclusion of the ethical principles provided their wording is improved. Some participants have argued that they should be listed in a different order so as not to suggest that 'respect for persons' takes priority over the other principles.

In the revised Guidelines it will be made very clear that these principles are not listed in any order of priority. Since these principles have equal moral force, no one of them has priority over any of the others.

The purpose of having principles which, in the abstract, have equal moral force is to provoke fruitful discussions about how to balance the requirements of these often competing principles in consideration of particular protocols. There will always be competition between considerations of distributive justice and, for example, respect for persons. Considerations of distributive justice often demand that we tell some people that they cannot have some of the things they want.

Several conferees voiced concern that the revised Guidelines should not appear to dissociate considerations of science and ethics. One component of the principle of beneficence is an obligation to maximize benefits to the collective; this obligation gives rise to the ethical requirements for sound scientific design and competent investigators, found in the Nuremberg Code and the Declaration of Helsinki.

In one of our sessions there was discussion of the competition between idealism and pragmatism in the development of guidelines. It was made clear that our Guidelines should point the way toward idealistic standards — what we hope will eventually evolve — with some pragmatic commentary stating what one expects while we are working in that direction. This point was made particularly well by Judith Miller in the report she gave on behalf of her working group. As she explained it, when we must compromise with the ideal we should recognize the need for compromise as a signal to take action to enhance the capacity of researchers and members of research ethics committees to more closely approximate the ideal. That subtlety may be difficult to capture in the form of guidelines but we should try.

Finally, I want to say that we have come a long way since Mexico City and Manila, the locations of the conferences that led to the development of the 1982 Guidelines. We have not only increased in number: we have increased remarkably in sophistication. The discussions at the meetings this week have been vastly different from those in either Manila or Mexico City. If all of the important things that have been said at this conference were to be incorporated in the revised Guidelines, they could easily become a rather lengthy book. I believe that the Guidelines should not be excessively detailed. They should not attempt either to anticipate or to rigidly control every contingency that could arise in the conduct of research involving human subjects. The Guidelines should provide guidance, a set of general principles which will facilitate the work of ethical review committees, encouraging them to make judgments and take decisions that are appropriate to the settings in which the research is to be conducted. Attempts to develop overly detailed and inflexible directives for behaviour would be counterproductive. Among other things, they would remove incentives for ethical review committee members to take responsibility for their decisions and to aspire to the ideals reflected in the Guidelines.

CLOSING OF THE CONFERENCE

F. Vilardell

Professor Bryant, Professor Levine, Members of CIOMS, Distinguished Guests, Ladies and Gentlemen:

It is certainly a great honour to bring this Twenty-Sixth CIOMS Conference to a close. During three days, nearly 150 participants from 35 very diverse countries have been working arduously on the documents prepared by the Steering Committee to facilitate the revision of the 1982 edition of the International Guidelines for Biomedical Research involving Human Subjects. The main themes of the group discussions have been individual consent and the agreement of communities to participate in research; the problems raised by disadvantaged and vulnerable populations; the establishment of national and local ethical committees; the review of research sponsored by agencies from other countries and of multi-centre trials, especially in the developing countries; and the obligations of sponsors, including access of the participating subjects to the benefits of the research and compensation for any harm arising from participation in research.

In the past 10 years new ethical aspects of research have emerged, such as those of molecular genetics and biology and epidemiology. Many problems are still far from solved, such as research on embryos or fetal tissue, investigations in the elderly and in particularly vulnerable individuals, including patients recovering in emergency wards and in intensive care units.

As a practising physician, personally involved in clinical research and in the ethical review of research protocols, I can only expect that the final revised version of the guidelines will be an indispensable tool for all those interested in the protection of human rights who are involved in clinical research, in the so-called developed countries as much as in the developing ones, as we can all identify particular groups of underprivileged and vulnerable populations in all countries without exception.

I hope that the ethical awakening which we are now witnessing in most parts of the world will contribute to disseminating the awareness of the value of these Guidelines, which are the result of strenuous effort on the part of a group of most dedicated people.

May I thank the untiring chairpersons of the Conference, Professors Bryant and Levine, and the other members of the Conference Programme Committee, B.M. Dickens, F. Gutteridge and D.L. Heymann. Special thanks must be given to Professor Gostin and to Ms Jordan for their valuable contribution in preparing An Annotated Guide to Ethical Review of Research on Human Subjects, as well to Mr. S.S. Fluss and his co-authors for their outstanding report on the legislation on ethical research around the world. I should like to acknowledge the invaluable help of the CIOMS secretariat, Ms K. Chalaby-Amsler and Ms C. Dubendorfer, as well as the disinterested assistance of Mrs E. Bankowski. Last but not least, may I express my gratitude for the essential contribution of Dr Z. Bankowski, CIOMS Secretary-General, in the preparation, the organization and the final success of the Conference.

The XXVIth CIOMS Conference is now officially closed.

LIST OF PARTICIPANTS

Abdussalam, M. Bundesgesundheitsamt, Berlin, Germany
Abrams, M. Department of Health, London, England
Andersen, B. Ministry of Health, Copenhagen, Denmark
André, A. Académie Royale de Médecine de Belgique, Liège, Belgium
Andreatti, T. Saint-Siège, Mission permanente, Geneva, Switzerland
Antezana, F.S. Action Programme on Essential Drugs, World Health Organization, Geneva, Switzerland
Bacou, J. Institut des Sciences de la Santé, Paris, France
Bankowski, Z. Council for International Organizations of Medical Sciences, Geneva, Switzerland
Banuelos, J.A. International Society for Burn Injuries, Barcelona, Spain
Belchior, M. Council for International Organizations of Medical Sciences, Rio de Janeiro, Brazil
Belsey, M. Maternal and Child Health and Family Planning, World Health Organization, Geneva, Switzerland
Berentey, G. Federation of Hungarian Medical Societies, Budapest, Hungary
Bhamarapravati, N. Mahidol University, Bangkok, Thailand
Bjarnason, O. Ministry of Health and Social Security, Department of Hygiene, Occupational Safety and Health, Reykjavik, Iceland
Blasi, W. International Clinical Research, F. Hoffmann-La Roche, Basel, Switzerland
Brockway, G.M. Mies, Vaud, Switzerland
Bryant, J.H. Department of Community Health Sciences, The Aga Khan University, Karachi, Pakistan
Bulyzhenkov, V. Hereditary Diseases Programme, World Health Organization, Geneva, Switzerland
Byk, C. Committee on Bioethics, Council of Europe, Paris, France
Capron, A.M. The Law Center, University of Southern California, Los Angeles, California, U.S.A.
Chrusciel, T. Chamber of Physicians, Warsaw, Poland
Chrzanowski, R. Swiss Public Health Institute, Lausanne, Switzerland
Cone, M. Scientific Affairs, International Federation of Pharmaceutical Manufacturers Associations, Geneva, Switzerland
Cook, R.J. International Human Rights Programme, University of Toronto, Faculty of Law, Toronto, Canada
Davidson, D.E. Special Programme for Research and Training in Tropical Diseases, World Health Organization, Geneva, Switzerland
Davies, A.M. School of Public Health, Jerusalem, Israel
Dickens, B.M. University of Toronto, Faculty of Law, Toronto, Canada
Dixon, P.H. World Veterans Federation, Surrey, England

Dowlati, Y. Ministry of Health and Education, Teheran, Iran

Dunne, J.F. Secretariat Committee on Research Involving Human Subjects, World Health Organization, Geneva, Switzerland

Fluss, S.S. Health Legislation, World Health Organization, Geneva, Switzerland

Fournier, D. World Association for Psychosocial Rehabilitation, Geneva, Switzerland

Gabr, M. Faculty of Medicine, University of Cairo, Cairo, Egypt

Gallagher, J. Council for International Organizations of Medical Sciences, Geneva, Switzerland

Gautier, E. Medicus Mundi, Colombier, Vaud, Switzerland

Gevers, J.K.M. Royal Netherlands Academy of Arts and Sciences, Amsterdam, Netherlands

Gezairy, H.A. Director, Regional Office for the Eastern Mediterranean, World Health Organization, Alexandria, Egypt

Gillon, R. Imperial College of Science, Technology and Medicine, and St Mary's Hospital Medical School, University of London, London, England

Glick, S. Center for Medical Education, Faculty of Health Sciences, Ben-Gurion University of the Negev, Beer-Sheva, Israel

Goon, E. Development of Human Resources for Health, World Health Organization, Geneva, Switzerland

Gornicki, B. Federation of Polish Medical Societies, Warsaw, Poland

Grahn, G. International Society of Nurses in Cancer Care, Lund, Sweden

Grodin, M.A. Law, Medicine and Ethics Program, School of Public Health and Medicine, Boston, Massachusetts, U.S.A.

Gromb, S. Université de Bordeaux, Pessac, France

Grossklaus, D. Federal Health Office, Berlin, Germany

Guillod, O. Geneva, Switzerland

Guldberg, H.C. Ethical Review Committee-Norway, University of Trondheim Medical School, Trondheim, Norway

Gutteridge, F. Council for International Organizations of Medical Sciences, Geneva, Switzerland

Gyarfas, I. Cardiovascular Diseases, World Health Organization, Geneva, Switzerland

Hachen, H.-J. International Rehabilitation Medicine Association; World Federation of Spine Surgeons and Spondyliatrists, Geneva, Switzerland

Hals, A. Medical Ethics Review Board, University of Trondheim Faculty of Medicine, Trondheim, Norway

Hanson, G. Radiation Medicine, World Health Organization, Geneva, Switzerland

Hapsara, H. Division of Epidemiological Surveillance and Health Situation and Trend Assessment, World Health Organization, Geneva, Switzerland

Hasan, Z. Behavioural Science Division, Baqai Medical College, Karachi, Pakistan

Hoffenberg, R. Wolfson College, Oxford, England

Hole, O. Regional Committee for Medical Research Ethics, Oslo, Norway

Hu, Ching-Li. Assistant Director-General, World Health Organization, Geneva, Switzerland

Idanpaan-Heikkila, J. Drug Management and Policies, World Health Organization, Geneva, Switzerland

Jardel, J.-P. Assistant Director-General, World Health Organization, Geneva, Switzerland

Johannisson, E. International Federation of Fertility Societies, Geneva, Switzerland

Jordan, L.C. Somerville, Massachusetts, U.S.A.

Kallings, L.O. Global Programme on AIDS, World Health Organization, Geneva, Switzerland

Karjalainen, S. National Agency for Welfare and Health, Helsinki, Finland

Kaushik, V. Institute of Philosophy, Academy of Sciences, Moscow, Russia

Khan, K.S. Department of Community Health Sciences, The Aga Khan University, Karachi, Pakistan

Kimura, R. Professor, School of Human Sciences, Waseda University, Tokorozawa, Japan; Kennedy Institute of Ethics, Georgetown University, Washington, D.C., U.S.A.

Kostrzewski, J. State Institute of Hygiene, Department of Epidemiology, Warsaw, Poland

Last, J.M. International Epidemiological Association; Faculty of Medicine, University of Ottawa, Ottawa, Canada

Legemaate, J. Royal Dutch Medical Association, National Committee on AIDS Control, Maarssen, Netherlands

Lepes, T. Department of Microbiology, Ethical Committee, Medical Faculty, Novi Sad, Ex-Yugoslavia

Leung-Nakatani, T. International Society of Chemotherapy, Oslo, Norway

Levaux, P. National Fund for Scientific Research, Brussels, Belgium

Levine, R.J. School of Medicine, Yale University, New Haven, Connecticut, U.S.A.

Lojacono, G. Consultà di Bioetica-Italy, Rome, Italy

Lommel, H. World Association of Societies of Pathology (Anatomic and Clinical), Leverkusen, Germany

Lopukhin, Y. Research Institute for Physico-Chemical Medicine, Moscow, Russia

Lowrance, W. International Medical Benefit/Risk Foundation, Geneva, Switzerland

Lumholtz, B. Sandoz Pharma Ltd., Basel, Switzerland

Lwin, U. Myint. Department of Medical Research, Ministry of Health, Yangon, Myanmar

Mansourian, B. Office of Research Promotion and Development, World Health Organization, Geneva, Switzerland

Mariner, W.K. Boston University School of Public Health, Boston, Massachusetts, U.S.A.

Marshall, T.D. Medical Research Council of Canada, Ottawa, Canada

Mattheis, R. Senatsverwaltung für Gesundheit u. Soziales, Berlin, Germany

Maurice, N.P. Corporate Human Research Quality Assurance, Ciba-Geigy, Basel, Switzerland

McCarthy, Ch. Former Director, Office for Protection from Research Risks, National Institutes of Health, Bethesda, Maryland, U.S.A.

Merritt-Lachenal, M. World Federation for Mental Health, Geneva, Switzerland

Miller, J. National Council on Bioethics in Human Research, Ottawa, Canada

Mork, T. Directorate of Health, Oslo, Norway

Motzel, C. Medical Women's International Association, Cologne, Germany

Napalkov, N.P. Assistant Director-General, World Health Organization, Geneva, Switzerland

Ngugi, E. Department of Community Health and Medical Microbiology, University of Nairobi, Nairobi, Kenya

Nicholson, R.H. Bulletin of Medical Ethics, London, England

Nyquist, I. Ethical Committee, Oslo, Norway

Oguisso, T. International Council of Nurses, Geneva, Switzerland

Osuntokun, B.O. University of Ibadan Department of Medicine, Ibadan, Nigeria

Papavassilliou, J. International Congresses of Tropical Medicine and Malaria, Athens, Greece

Perez, M.I. Saint-Siège, Mission permanente, Geneva, Switzerland

Perriens, J. Institute of Tropical Medicine, Antwerp, Belgium

Piga, A. Health Legislation, Regional Office for Europe, World Health Organization, Copenhagen, Denmark

Pinet, G. Legal Counsel, World Health Organization, Geneva, Switzerland

Qiu Ren-Zong. Institute of Philosophy, Chinese Academy of Social Sciences, Beijing, People's Republic of China

Rabbee, J.A. Health Services, Government of Bangladesh, Dacca, Bangladesh

Ram, E. World Vision International, Monrovia, California, U.S.A.

Reinstein, J. World Federation of Proprietary Medicine Manufacturers, London, England

Relación, J.R. Committee on Ethics, Asia-Oceania Federation of Obstetrics & Gynecology, Manila, Philippines

Rentchnick, P. Médecine et Hygiène, Geneva, Switzerland

Rifka, G. Eastern Mediterranean Liaison Office, World Health Organization, Geneva, Switzerland

Riis, P. National Scientific-Ethical Committee of Denmark, Copenhagen, Denmark

Roscam-Abbing, H. Ministry of Health, Rijswijk, Netherlands

Rudowski, W. Medical Section, Polish Academy of Sciences, Warsaw, Poland

Rushton, A. ICI Pharmaceuticals, Medical Research Department, Macclesfield, England

Rutishauser, W. International Society and Federation of Cardiology, Geneva, Switzerland

Saracci, R. International Agency for Research on Cancer, Lyon, France

Schersten, T. Swedish Medical Research Council, Stockholm, Sweden

Scott, R.M. Expanded Programme on Immunization, World Health Organization, Geneva, Switzerland

de Scoville, A. Académie royale de Médecine de Belgique, Brussels, Belgium

Siest, G. International Federation of Clinical Chemistry, Nancy, France

Simoen, M.-J. National Fund for Scientific Research, Brussels, Belgium

Slade, D. International Association of Medical Laboratory Technologists, Bath, England

Sleep, J. International Confederation of Midwives, Eversley, Hants, U.K.

Soberon, G. Fundación Mexicana para la Salud, Mexico City, Mexico

Solbakk, J.H. The Norwegian Research Council for Science and the Humanities, Oslo, Norway

Soutoul, E. Centre hospitalier régional et universitaire, Rennes, France

Sprumont, D. Séminaire de Droit constitutionnel, Université de Fribourg, Fribourg, Switzerland

Stober, J.A. Environmental Health, World Health Organization, Geneva, Switzerland

Strasser, Th. World Hypertension League, Geneva, Switzerland

Straume, B. Regional Board for Medical Research Ethics, University of Tromsø, Tromsø, Norway

Stutz-Steiger, T. Federal Office of Public Health, Medical and Pharmaceutical Division, Berne, Switzerland

Sureau, C. International Federation of Gynecology and Obstetrics, Paris, France

de Sweemer-Ba, C. Centre de Recherches pour le Développement international, Dakar, Senegal

Szczerban, J. Office of Research Promotion and Development, World Health Organization, Geneva, Switzerland

Thuriaux, M.C. Strengthening of Epidemiological and Statistical Services, World Health Organization, Geneva, Switzerland

Trasco Michel, M. Centro de Bioetica U. Catolica Sacro Cuore, Rome, Italy

Tubiana, M. Former Director, Institut Gustave-Roussy, Villejuif, France

Uehara, N. Department of International Cooperation, National Medical Center, Tokyo, Japan

Vandvik, B. Ethical Committee, Oslo, Norway

Varnai, F. Federation of Hungarian Medical Societies, Budapest, Hungary

Venulet, J. Council for International Organizations of Medical Sciences, Geneva, Switzerland

Vickers, M. World Federation of Societies of Anaesthesiology, Cardiff, U.K.

Vilardell, F. Council for International Organizations of Medical Sciences; World Organization of Gastroenterology, Barcelona, Spain

Vizi, S. Scientific and Research Ethics Committee, Hungarian Health Science Board, Budapest, Hungary

de Wachter, M.A.M. Institute for Bioethics, Maastricht, Netherlands

Wells, F. Association of the British Pharmaceutical Industry (ABPI), London, England

Wilson, E.W. Special Programme of Research, Development and Research Training in Human Reproduction, World Health Organization, Geneva, Switzerland

Wint, U Maung. Yangon General Hospital, Department of Health, Yangon, Myanmar

Winther, F. Rikshospitalet, Oslo, Norway

Wynen, A. World Medical Association, Ferney-Voltaire, France

Zakopoulos, Athenagoras. Metropolitan of Fokidos, Greek Orthodox Church, Amfissa, Fokida, Greece

Zhang Ju. Department of Social Sciences, Peking Union Medical College, Beijing, People's Republic of China

International Ethical Guidelines
for
Biomedical Research
Involving Human Subjects

Prepared by the Council for International
Organizations of Medical Sciences (CIOMS)
in collaboration with
the World Health Organization (WHO)

Geneva
1993

CONTENTS

ACKNOWLEDGEMENTS

The Council for International Organizations of Medical Sciences (CIOMS) acknowledges the very substantial contribution, financial and technical, of the World Health Organization Global Programme on AIDS to the preparation of *International Ethical Guidelines for Research Involving Human Subjects*. The two other Special Programmes of the World Health Organization — on Research, Development and Research Training in Human Reproduction, and for Research and Training in Tropical Diseases — also gave valuable support. CIOMS acknowledges also with much appreciation the financial contributions of the Sandoz Foundation in the United States of America and the International Development Research Centre of Canada.

Of the many individuals who contributed to the preparation of the Guidelines, the following merit special acknowledgement: Professor Robert J. Levine who was Co-Chairman of the CIOMS Steering Committee and the Conference on Ethics and Research on Human Subjects — International Guidelines, and provided invaluable assistance from the inception of the project, particularly in the preparation of several drafts and the final text of the Guidelines; Professor John H. Bryant who co-chaired the Conference and the Steering Committee, and whose wise counsel was available throughout; Professor Bernard M. Dickens and Mr Richard Kelly who prepared the first draft of the Guidelines; Professor Lawrence O. Gostin, for his part in preparing An Annotated Guide to Ethical Review, which was used in the preparation of the Guidelines; and Professors Mohamed Abdussalam, Wendy Mariner and Benjamin O. Osuntokun, Mr Frank Gutteridge, Mr Sev S. Fluss and Dr Michel Thuriaux, who contributed actively from the beginning. Special thanks go to Dr James Gallagher for his contribution to the final drafting and editing of the Guidelines, and to Mrs Kathryn Chalaby-Amsler for her invaluable secretarial assistance.

BACKGROUND NOTE

Advances in biomedical science and technology, and their application in the practice of medicine, are provoking some anxiety among the public and confronting society with new ethical problems. Society is expressing concern about what it fears would be abuses in scientific investigation and biomedical technology. This is understandable in view of the methodology of biomedical experimental research. Investigation begins with the construction of hypotheses and these are then tested in laboratories and with experimental animals. For the findings to be clinically useful, experiments must be performed on human subjects, and, even though carefully designed, such research entails some risk to the subjects. This risk is justified not by any personal benefit to the researcher or the research institution, but rather by its benefit to the human subjects involved, and its potential contribution to human knowledge, to the relief of suffering or to the prolongation of life.

Society devises measures to protect against possible abuses. The first international code of ethics for research involving human subjects — the Nuremberg Code — was a response to the atrocities committed by Nazi research physicians, revealed at the Nuremberg War Crimes Trials. Thus it was to prevent any repetition by physicians of such attacks on the rights and welfare of human beings that human-research ethics came into being. The Nuremberg Code, issued in 1947, laid down the standards for carrying out human experimentation, emphasizing the subject's voluntary consent. In 1964 the World Medical Association took an important step further to reassure society: it adopted the Declaration of Helsinki, most recently revised in 1989, which lays down ethical guidelines for research involving human subjects. In 1966 the United Nations General Assembly adopted the International Covenant on Civil and Political Rights, which entered into force in 1976, and which states (Article 7): *"No one shall be subjected to torture or to cruel, inhuman or degrading treatment or punishment. In particular, no one shall be subjected without his free consent to medical or scientific experimentation"*. It is through this statement that society expresses the fundamental human value that is held to govern all research involving human subjects — the protection of the rights and welfare of all human subjects of scientific experimentation.

In the late 1970s, in view of the special circumstances of developing countries in regard to the applicability of the Nuremberg Code and the Declaration of Helsinki, the Council for International Organizations of Medical Sciences (CIOMS) and the World Health Organization (WHO) undertook a further examination of these matters, and in 1982 issued *Proposed International Guidelines for Biomedical Research Involving Human Subjects*. The purpose of the *Proposed Guidelines* was to indicate how the ethical principles that should guide the conduct of biomedical research involving human subjects, as set forth in the Declaration of Helsinki, could be effectively applied, particularly in developing countries, given their socioeconomic circumstances, laws and regulations, and executive and administrative arrangements.

Proposed Guidelines received extensive distribution and, according to a later survey, went into use widely throughout the world, providing valuable ethical guidance in biomedical research involving human subjects. Survey respondents and other users indicated also that the guidelines should be reviewed with particular reference to the ethical issues raised by large-scale trials of vaccines and drugs, transnational research, and experimentation involving vulnerable population groups. A particular indication for their revision was the prospect of field trials of vaccines and drugs to control AIDS. Moreover, in recent years, many people, in developed and developing countries alike, have begun to see the beneficial and not only the threatening aspects of research involving human subjects; indeed such research, particularly related to innovative therapy trials, is now actively sought by potential beneficiaries. For some, participation in research is the only way they can gain access to valuable new treatment or even general medical care; for others, it is the means by which scientists will discover new knowledge that may lead to the prevention or treatment or even elimination of certain categories of disease and disability.

In these circumstances CIOMS undertook, in collaboration with WHO, the revision of the guidelines, setting up a steering committee to guide the process. The Steering Committee decided that in the revision special attention should be paid to epidemiological studies, owing to the importance of epidemiology, particularly for public health, and to the need for international guidelines for ethical review of such studies. In the event, it was determined that this need would be best met by a separate publication, and the result was the issuing by CIOMS in 1991 of *International Guidelines for Ethical Review of Epidemiological Studies*. The preparation of the epidemiological guidelines contributed materially to the revision of the 1982 guidelines.

After extensive consultation the first draft of the revised guidelines was prepared by a group of consultants, reviewed and amended by the Steering Committee, and presented to the CIOMS Conference on Ethics and Research on Human Subjects — International Guidelines, held in Geneva in February 1992. At the conference it was examined and discussed by some 150 participants from both developed and developing countries, including representatives of ministries of health and medical and other health-related disciplines, health policy-makers, ethicists, philosophers and lawyers.

The draft guidelines were revised to reflect the consensus of the conference, but with due regard to minority points of view. The revised draft was then sent for comment to the conference participants, to international associations, and to medical research councils and other interested bodies and institutions in both developed and developing countries. The final text duly reflects the comments received. It has been endorsed by the WHO Global Advisory Committee on Health Research and the Executive Committee of CIOMS, which have recommended its publication and wide distribution.

The text consists of a statement of general ethical principles, a preamble and 15 guidelines, with an introduction, and a brief account of earlier ethical declaration and guidelines. Each guideline is followed by a commentary.

The guidelines reflect the paramount ethical concern for vigilance in protecting the rights and welfare of research subjects and of vulnerable individuals or groups being considered as prospective subjects. Like the original (1982) guidelines, the revised guidelines are designed to be of use, particularly to developing countries, in defining national policies on the ethics of biomedical research, applying ethical standards in local circumstances, and establishing or redefining adequate mechanisms for ethical review of research involving human subjects.

Certain areas of research do not receive special mention in these guidelines; they include human genetic research, embryo and fetal research, and fetal tissue research. These represent research areas in rapid evolution and in various respects controversial. The Steering Committee considered that since there is not universal agreement on all the ethical issues raised by these research areas it would be premature to try to cover them in the present guidelines.

The mere formulation of ethical guidelines for biomedical research involving human subjects will hardly resolve all the moral doubts that can arise in association with such research, but the guidelines can at least draw the attention of investigators, sponsors and ethical review committees to the need to consider carefully the ethical implications of research protocols and the conduct of research, and thus conduce to high scientific and ethical standards of research.

Comments on the Guidelines are welcome, and will be taken into account in future revisions. They should be addressed to:

Zbigniew Bankowski, M.D.
Secretary-General
Council for International Organizations of Medical Sciences
c/o World Health Organization
CH-1211 Geneva 27, Switzerland

INTRODUCTION

As a result of collaboration on research ethics between the World Health Organization (WHO) and the Council for International Organizations of Medical Sciences (CIOMS), CIOMS published in 1982 *Proposed International Guidelines for Biomedical Research Involving Human Subjects*. The purpose of the Guidelines was to indicate how the fundamental ethical principles that guide the conduct of biomedical research involving human subjects, as set forth in the World Medical Association's Declaration of Helsinki, could be applied effectively, particularly in developing countries, taking into account culture, socioeconomic circumstances, national laws, and executive and administrative arrangements.

The Guidelines were distributed to ministries of health, medical research councils, medical faculties, non-governmental organizations, research-based pharmaceutical companies, other interested bodies and medical journals. Comments on the Guidelines and suggestions for amendments were received from many sources. Also CIOMS carried out a questionnaire survey, with due representation of developing countries and all six WHO regions. The responses indicated that biomedical scientists in many countries appreciated the ethical guidance the Guidelines provided, particularly in assuring the validity of informed consent and otherwise protecting the rights and welfare of research subjects; they suggested also various areas for amendment and review.

In the years that followed, it became obvious that a number of developing countries were finding the Guidelines helpful in setting up their own arrangements for independent ethical review of proposed biomedical research projects but that certain changes in emphasis were needed.

Also since 1982 there have been considerable advances in medical sciences and biotechnology, and the potential of human biomedical research has continued to expand. The AIDS epidemic, particularly the need to carry out vaccine and drug trials, has raised ethical questions that were not foreseen when the Declaration of Helsinki was formulated, or even only ten years ago when the CIOMS Guidelines were issued. In some countries people at risk of HIV infection have claimed a right to access to clinical research and to incompletely tested new treatments. In some societies, the deliberate exclusion from research of women who are pregnant or capable of becoming pregnant, to avoid risk to the fetus, has begun to be questioned on the grounds that it deprives such women of benefits and denies them their right to decide for themselves whether to take part in research. Similarly, the growth of geriatric medicine and geriatric pharmacology has created pressure for the inclusion of elderly people in medical research for their own benefit.

International and intercultural collaborative research has increased considerably and involves developing countries, many of which have yet a very limited capacity for independent review of research proposals submitted by either external sponsors and investigators or their own research workers.

Finally, there is some concern about biomedical research involving human subjects being regarded as a benefit to its subjects and to society, rather than only as a source of risk to its subjects. Many people regard this claim with some apprehension in case research will be undertaken or promoted without adequate justification and secure safeguards of the rights and welfare of the research subjects.

In all these circumstances it appeared timely to revise the 1982 Guidelines, with a view to reaffirming in today's conditions their original purpose — the protection of the rights and welfare of human subjects of biomedical research.

INTERNATIONAL DECLARATIONS AND GUIDELINES

The first international document on the ethics of research, the Nuremberg Code, was promulgated in 1947 as a consequence of the trial of physicians who had conducted atrocious experiments on unconsenting prisoners and detainees during the second world war. The Code, designed to protect the integrity of the research subject, sets out conditions for the ethical conduct of research involving human subjects, emphasizing the human subject's "voluntary consent" to research.

To give the Universal Declaration of Human Rights, adopted by the United Nations General Assembly in 1948, legal as well as moral force, the General Assembly of the United Nations adopted in 1966 the International Covenant on Civil and Political Rights, of which Article 7 states *"No one shall be subjected to torture or to cruel, inhuman or degrading treatment or punishment. In particular, no one shall be subjected without his free consent to medical or scientific experimentation."*

The Declaration of Helsinki, promulgated in 1964 by the World Medical Association, is the fundamental document in the field of ethics in biomedical research and has had considerable influence on the formulation of international, regional and national legislation and codes of conduct. The Declaration, revised in Tokyo in 1975, in Venice in 1983, and again in Hong Kong in 1989, is a comprehensive international statement of the ethics of research involving human subjects. It sets out ethical guidelines for physicians engaged in both clinical and non-clinical biomedical research, and provides among its rules for informed consent of subjects and ethical review of the research protocol. The Declaration of Helsinki is appended (Annex 1).

The publication in 1982 of *Proposed International Guidelines for Biomedical Research Involving Human Subjects* was a logical develop-ment of the Declaration of Helsinki. As stated in the Introduction of that publication, the Guidelines were intended to indicate how the ethical principles embodied in the Declaration could be effectively applied in developing countries. The text explained the application of established ethical principles to biomedical research involving human subjects and drew attention to new ethical issues arising in the period that preceded their publication. The present publication, *International Ethical Guidelines for Biomedical Research Involving Human Subjects,* supersedes the 1982 *Proposed International Guidelines.*

CIOMS and WHO have continued to work together to provide ethical guidance for research involving human subjects. One important outcome of this cooperation has been *International Guidelines for Ethical Review of Epidemiological Studies,* published by CIOMS in 1991, intended to assist investigators and institutions as well as regional and national authorities in setting and maintaining standards for the ethical review of epidemiological studies.

GENERAL ETHICAL PRINCIPLES

All research involving human subjects should be conducted in accordance with three basic ethical principles, namely respect for persons, beneficence and justice. It is generally agreed that these principles, which in the abstract have equal moral force, guide the conscientious preparation of proposals for scientific studies. In varying circumstances they may be expressed differently and given different moral weight, and their application may lead to different decisions or courses of action. The present guidelines are directed at the application of these principles to research involving human subjects.

Respect for persons incorporates at least two fundamental ethical considerations, namely:
  a) respect for autonomy, which requires that those who are capable of deliberation about their personal choices should be treated with respect for their capacity for self-determination; and
  b) protection of persons with impaired or diminished autonomy, which requires that those who are dependent or vulnerable be afforded security against harm or abuse.

Beneficence refers to the ethical obligation to maximize benefits and to minimize harms and wrongs. This principle gives rise to norms requiring that the risks of research be reasonable in the light of the expected benefits, that the research design be sound, and that the investigators be competent both to conduct the research and to safeguard the welfare of the research subjects. Beneficence further proscribes the deliberate infliction of harm on persons; this aspect of beneficence is sometimes expressed as a separate principle, **non-maleficence** (do no harm).

Justice refers to the ethical obligation to treat each person in accordance with what is morally right and proper, to give each person what is due to him or her. In the ethics of research involving human subjects the principle refers primarily to **distributive justice,** which requires the equitable distribution of both the burdens and the benefits of participation in research. Differences in distribution of burdens and benefits are justifiable only if they are based on morally relevant distinctions between persons; one such distinction is vulnerability. "Vulnerability" refers to a substantial incapacity to protect one's own interests owing to such impediments as lack of capability to give informed consent, lack of alternative means of obtaining medical care or other expensive necessities, or being a junior or subordinate member of a hierarchical group. Accordingly, special provisions must be made for the protection of the rights and welfare of vulnerable persons.

PREAMBLE

The term "research" refers to a class of activities designed to develop or contribute to generalizable knowledge. Generalizable knowledge consists of theories, principles or relationships, or the accumulation of information on which they are based, that can be corroborated by accepted scientific methods of observation and inference. In the present context "research" includes both medical and behavioural studies pertaining to human health. Usually "research" is modified by the adjective "biomedical" to indicate that the reference is to health-related research.

Progress in medical care and disease prevention depends upon an understanding of physiological and pathological processes or epidemiological findings, and requires at some time research involving human subjects. The collection, analysis and interpretation of information obtained from research involving human beings contribute significantly to the improvement of human health.

Research involving human subjects includes that undertaken together with patient care (clinical research) and that undertaken on patients or other subjects, or with data pertaining to them, solely to contribute to generalizable knowledge (non-clinical biomedical research). Research is defined as "clinical" if one or more of its components is designed to be diagnostic, prophylactic or therapeutic for the individual subject of the research. Invariably, in clinical research, there are also components designed not to be diagnostic, prophylactic or therapeutic for the subject; examples include the administration of placebos and the performance of laboratory tests in addition to those required to serve the purposes of medical care. Hence the term "clinical research" is used here rather than "therapeutic research".

Research involving human subjects includes:
- studies of a physiological, biochemical or pathological process, or of the response to a specific intervention — whether physical, chemical or psychological — in healthy subjects or patients;
- controlled trials of diagnostic, preventive or therapeutic measures in larger groups of persons, designed to demonstrate a specific generalizable response to these measures against a background of individual biological variation;

11

- studies designed to determine the consequences for individuals and communities of specific preventive or therapeutic measures; and
- studies concerning human health-related behaviour in a variety of circumstances and environments.

Research involving human subjects may employ either observation or physical, chemical or psychological intervention; it may also either generate records or make use of existing records containing biomedical or other information about individuals who may or may not be identifiable from the records or information. The use of such records and the protection of the confidentiality of data obtained from those records are discussed in *International Guidelines for Ethical Review of Epidemiological Studies* (CIOMS, 1991).

Research involving human subjects includes also research in which environmental factors are manipulated in a way that could affect incidentally-exposed individuals. Research is defined in broad terms in order to embrace field studies of pathogenic organisms and toxic chemicals under investigation for health-related purposes.

Research involving human subjects is to be distinguished from the practice of medicine, public health and other forms of health care, which is designed to contribute directly to the health of individuals or communities. Prospective subjects may find it confusing when research and practice are to be conducted simultaneously, as when research is designed to obtain new information about the efficacy of a drug or other therapeutic, diagnostic or preventive modality.

Research involving human subjects should be carried out only by, or strictly supervised by, suitably qualified and experienced investigators and in accordance with a protocol that clearly states: the aim of the research; the reasons for proposing that it involve human subjects; the nature and degree of any known risks to the subjects; the sources from which it is proposed to recruit subjects; and the means proposed for ensuring that subjects' consent will be adequately informed and voluntary. The protocol should be scientifically and ethically appraised by one or more suitably constituted review bodies, independent of the investigators.

New vaccines and medicinal drugs, before being approved for general use, must be tested on human subjects in clinical trials; such trials, which constitute a substantial part of all research involving human subjects, are described in Annex 2.

THE GUIDELINES

Informed Consent of Subjects

Guideline 1: Individual informed consent

For all biomedical research involving human subjects, the investigator must obtain the informed consent of the prospective subject or, in the case of an individual who is not capable of giving informed consent, the proxy consent of a properly authorized representative.

Commentary on Guideline 1

General considerations. Informed consent is consent given by a competent individual who has received the necessary information; who has adequately understood the information; and who, after considering the information, has arrived at a decision without having been subjected to coercion, undue influence or inducement, or intimidation.

Informed consent is based on the principle that competent individuals are entitled to choose freely whether to participate in research. Informed consent protects the individual's freedom of choice and respects the individual's autonomy.

In itself, informed consent is an imperfect safeguard for the individual, and it must always be complemented by independent ethical review of research proposals. Moreover, many individuals, including young children, many adults with severe mental or behavioural disorders, and many persons who are totally unfamiliar with modern medical concepts, are limited in their capacity to give adequate informed consent. Because their consent could imply passive and uncomprehending participation, investigators must on no account presume that consent given by such vulnerable individuals is valid, without the prior approval of an independent ethical-review body. When an individual is incapable of making an informed decision whether to participate in research, the investigator must obtain the proxy consent of the individual's legal guardian or other duly authorized representative.

When the research design involves no more than minimal risk — that is, risk that is no more likely and not greater than that attached to routine medical or psychological examination — and it is not practicable to obtain informed consent from each subject (for example, where the research involves only excerpting data from subjects' records) the ethical review committee may waive some or all of the elements of informed consent. Investigators should never initiate research involving human subjects without obtaining each subject's informed consent, unless they have received explicit approval to do so from an ethical review committee.

Guideline 2: Essential information for prospective research subjects

Before requesting an individual's consent to participate in research, the investigator must provide the individual with the following information, in language that he or she is capable of understanding:

- **that each individual is invited to participate as a subject in research, and the aims and methods of the research;**
- **the expected duration of the subject's participation;**
- **the benefits that might reasonably be expected to result to the subject or to others as an outcome of the research;**
- **any foreseeable risks or discomfort to the subject, associated with participation in the research;**
- **any alternative procedures or courses of treatment that might be as advantageous to the subject as the procedure or treatment being tested;**
- **the extent to which confidentiality of records in which the subject is identified will be maintained;**
- **the extent of the investigator's responsibility, if any, to provide medical services to the subject;**
- **that therapy will be provided free of charge for specified types of research-related injury;**
- **whether the subject or the subject's family or dependants will be compensated for disability or death resulting from such injury; and**
- **that the individual is free to refuse to participate and will be free to withdraw from the research at any time without penalty or loss of benefits to which he or she would otherwise be entitled.**

Commentary on Guideline 2

Process. Obtaining informed consent is a process that is begun when initial contact is made with a prospective subject and continues throughout the course of the study. By informing the subjects, by repetition and explanation, by answering subjects' questions as they arise, and by assuring that each procedure is understood by each subject, the research team not only elicits the informed consent of subjects but also manifests deep respect for the dignity of the subjects.

Language. Informing the subject must not be simply a ritual recitation of the contents of a form. Rather, the investigator must convey the information in words that suit the individual's level of understanding.

The investigator must bear in mind that ability to understand the information necessary to give informed consent depends on the individual's maturity, intelligence, education and rationality.

Comprehension. The investigator must then ensure that the prospective subject has adequately understood the information. This obligation is the more serious as risk to the subject increases. In some instances the investigator might administer an oral or a written test to check whether the information has been adequately understood.

Benefits. In research designed to evaluate vaccines, drugs or other products, subjects should be told whether and how the product will be made available to them if it proves to be safe and effective. They should be told whether they will have continuing access to the product between the end of their participation in the research and the time of approval of the product for general distribution, and whether they will receive it free of charge or will be expected to pay for it.

Risks. In the case of complex research projects it may be neither feasible nor desirable to inform prospective subjects fully about every possible risk. However, they must be informed of all risks that a reasonable person would consider material to making a decision about whether to participate. An investigator's judgment about what risks are to be considered material should be reviewed and approved by the ethical review committee (see Guideline 3). Subjects who desire additional information should be afforded an opportunity to ask questions.

The investigator's responsibility for medical care. If the investigator is a physician, the subject must be told clearly whether the investigator will act only as an investigator or as both an investigator and a physician to the subject. However, an investigator who agrees to act as physician-investigator undertakes all of the legal and ethical responsibilities of the subject's primary-care physician. In such a case, if the subject withdraws from the research owing to complications related to the research or in the exercise of the right to withdraw without loss of benefit, the physician has an obligation to continue to provide medical care to the subject, or to see that the subject receives the necessary care in the community or district health-care system, or to offer assistance in finding another physician.

If the investigator is to act only as an investigator, the subject must be advised to seek any necessary medical care, outside the context of the research.

Other considerations. For further details of the obligation to provide economic compensation in the event of death or disability resulting from specified types of research-related injury, see Guideline 13. For further discussion of confidentiality, see Guideline 12.

Guideline 3: Obligations of investigators regarding informed consent

The investigator has a duty to:
- **communicate to the prospective subject all the information necessary for adequately informed consent;**
- **give the prospective subject full opportunity and encouragement to ask questions;**
- **exclude the possibility of unjustified deception, undue influence and intimidation;**
- **seek consent only after the prospective subject has adequate knowledge of the relevant facts and of the consequences of participation, and has had sufficient opportunity to consider whether to participate;**
- **as a general rule, obtain from each prospective subject a signed form as evidence of informed consent; and**
- **renew the informed consent of each subject if there are material changes in the conditions or procedures of the research.**

Commentary on Guideline 3

Necessary information. The standards for communicating information as set forth in Guidelines 2 and 3 should be regarded as minimum. Other types of information that should be conveyed include the reasons for selecting prospective subjects (ordinarily because they either have certain diseases or have no apparent disease) and certain features of the research design (for example, randomization, double-blind, case-control), stated in language that the subjects can understand. Additional types of information that should be conveyed in some circumstances are suggested below in the commentaries on several other guidelines. In general the standard for communicating information is that any and all information that a reasonable person would consider material to reaching a decision about whether to consent should be communicated. Investigators and ethical review committees should determine together what should be communicated in connection with particular studies.

Opportunity to ask questions. The investigator must be prepared to answer all of the subject's questions relating to the proposed research. Any restriction of the subject's ability to ask questions and receive answers before or during the research undermines the validity of the informed consent.

Deception. Sometimes, to ensure valid research, subjects are deliberately misled. In biomedical research, deception mostly takes the form of withholding information about the purpose of procedures; for example, subjects in clinical trials are often not told the purpose of tests performed to monitor their compliance with the protocol, in case that if they knew their compliance was being monitored they would invalidate results by modifying their behaviour. In most such cases the prospective subjects are asked to consent to remain uninformed of the purpose of some procedures until the research is completed; in other cases, because a request for permission to withhold some information would jeopardize the validity of the research, prospective subjects are not made aware that some information has been withheld until the research is completed.

Telling lies to subjects is a tactic not commonly employed in biomedical research. However, social and behavioural scientists may deliberately misinform subjects to study their attitudes and behaviour; for example, scientists have pretended to be patients to study the behaviour of health-care professionals and patients in their natural settings.

Deception of the subject is not permissible in research projects that carry more than minimal risk of harm to the subject. When deception is indispensable to the methods of an experiment, the investigator must demonstrate to an ethical review committee that no other research method would suffice; that significant advances could result from the research; and that nothing has been withheld that, if divulged, would cause a reasonable person to refuse to participate. The ethical review committee with the investigator should determine whether and how deceived subjects should be informed of the deception upon completion of the research. Such informing, commonly called "debriefing", ordinarily entails explaining the reasons for the deception. A subject who disapproves of having been deceived is ordinarily offered an opportunity to refuse to allow the investigator to use information obtained from studying the subject.

Undue influence. The investigator should seek to exclude any undue influence on the subject. However, the borderline between justifiable persuasion and undue influence is imprecise. The investigator should not give the prospective subject any unjustifiable assurances about the benefits, risks or inconveniences of the research. An example of undue influence would be to induce a close relative or a community leader to influence a prospective subject's decision or to threaten to withhold health services. See also Guideline 4.

Intimidation. Intimidation in any form invalidates informed consent. Prospective subjects who are patients often depend upon the investigator for medical care, and the investigator has a certain credibility in their eyes. If the research protocol has a therapeutic component, the investigator's influence over them may be considerable. They may fear, for example, that refusal to participate would damage their relationship with the investigator. The investigator must assure prospective subjects that their decision on whether to participate will not affect the therapeutic relationship or any other benefits to which they are entitled.

Documentation of consent. Consent may be indicated in a number of ways. The subject may imply consent by his or her voluntary actions, express consent orally, or sign a consent form. As a general rule, the subject should sign a consent form, or, in the case of incompetence, a legal guardian or other duly authorized representative should do so. The ethical review committee may approve the waiving of the requirement of a signed consent form if the research carries no more than minimal risk and if the procedures to be used are only those for which signed consent forms are not customarily required outside the research context. Such waivers may also be approved when existence of a signed consent form would be an unjustified threat to the subjects' confidentiality. In some cases, particularly when the information is complicated, it is advisable to give subjects information sheets to retain; these may resemble consent forms in all respects except that subjects are not required to sign them.

Continuing consent. The initial consent should be renewed when material changes occur in the conditions or the procedures of the research. For example, new information may have come to light, either from the study or from outside the study, about the risks or benefits of therapies being tested or about alternatives to the therapies. Subjects should be given such information. In many clinical trials, data are not disclosed to subjects and investigators until the study is concluded. This is ethically acceptable if the data are monitored by a committee responsible for data and safety monitoring (see Guideline 14, page 40) and an ethical review committee has approved their non-disclosure.

Guideline 4: Inducement to participate

Subjects may be paid for inconvenience and time spent, and should be reimbursed for expenses incurred, in connection with their participation in research; they may also receive free medical services. However, the payments should not be so large or the medical services so extensive as to induce prospective subjects to consent to participate in the research against their better judgment ("undue inducement"). All payments, reimbursements and medical services to be provided to research subjects should be approved by an ethical review committee.

Commentary on Guideline 4

Acceptable recompense. Research subjects may have their transport and other expenses reimbursed and receive a modest allowance for inconvenience due to their participation in the research. Also,

18

investigators may provide them with medical services and the use of facilities, and perform procedures and tests free of charge, provided these are done in connection with the research.

Unacceptable recompense. Payments in money or in kind to research subjects should not be so large as to persuade them to take undue risks or volunteer against their better judgment. Payments or rewards that undermine a person's capacity to exercise free choice invalidate consent. It may be difficult to distinguish between suitable recompense and undue influence to participate in research. An unemployed person or a student may view promised recompense differently from an employed person. Someone without access to medical care may be unduly influenced to participate in research simply to receive such care. Therefore, monetary and in-kind recompense must be evaluated in the light of the traditions of the particular culture and population in which they are offered, to determine whether they constitute undue influence. The ethical review committee will ordinarily be the best judge of what constitutes reasonable material recompense in particular circumstances.

Incompetent persons. Incompetent persons may be vulnerable to exploitation for financial gain by guardians. A guardian asked to give proxy consent on behalf of an incompetent person should be offered no remuneration except a refund of out-of-pocket expenses.

Withdrawal from study. When a subject withdraws from research for reasons related to the study, or is withdrawn on health grounds, the investigator should pay the subject as if full participation had taken place. When a subject withdraws for any other reason, the investigator should pay in proportion to the amount of participation. An investigator who must remove a subject from the study for wilful noncompliance is entitled to withhold part or all of the payment.

Guideline 5: Research involving children

Before undertaking research involving children, the investigator must ensure that:
- **children will not be involved in research that might equally well be carried out with adults;**
- **the purpose of the research is to obtain knowledge relevant to the health needs of children;**
- **a parent or legal guardian of each child has given proxy consent;**
- **the consent of each child has been obtained to the extent of the child's capabilities;**
- **the child's refusal to participate in research must always be respected unless according to the research protocol the child would receive therapy for which there is no medically-acceptable alternative;**
- **the risk presented by interventions not intended to benefit the individual child-subject is low and commensurate with the importance of the knowledge to be gained; and**
- **interventions that are intended to provide therapeutic benefit are likely to be at least as advantageous to the individual child-subject as any available alternative.**

Commentary on Guideline 5

Justification of the involvement of children. The participation of children is indispensable for research into diseases of childhood and conditions to which children are particularly susceptible. The aims of the research should be relevant to the health needs of children.

Consent of the child. The willing cooperation of the child should be sought, after the child has been informed to the extent that the child's maturity and intelligence permit. The age at which a child becomes legally competent to give consent differs substantially from one jurisdiction to another; in some countries the "age of consent" established in their different provinces, states or other political subdivisions varies considerably. Often children who have not yet reached the legally established age of consent can understand the implications of informed consent and go through the necessary procedures; they can therefore knowingly agree to serve as research subjects. Such knowing agreement is insufficient to permit participation in research unless it is supplemented by the proxy consent of a parent, legal guardian or other duly authorized representative.

Older children who are capable of informed consent should be selected before younger children or infants, unless there are important scientific reasons related to age for involving younger children first. An objection by a child to taking part in research should always be respected even if the parent gives proxy consent, unless according to the research protocol the child would receive therapy for which there is no medically-acceptable alternative; in such a case parents or guardians may properly be authorized to override the objections of the child, particularly if the child is very young or immature.

Proxy consent of a parent or guardian. The investigator must obtain the proxy consent of the parent or guardian in accordance with local laws or established procedures. It may be assumed that children over the age of 13 years are usually capable of giving informed consent, but their consent must be complemented by the proxy consent of a parent or guardian, unless this is not required by local law.

Observation of research by parent. A parent or guardian who gives proxy consent for a child to participate in research should be given the opportunity to observe the research as it proceeds, so as to be able to withdraw the child from the research if the parent or guardian decides it is in the child's best interests to do so.

Psychological and medical support. Research involving children should be conducted in settings in which the child and the parent can obtain adequate medical and psychological support. As an additional protection for children, an investigator may, when possible, obtain the advice of a child's family physician or other health-care provider on matters concerning the child's involvement in the research.

Justification of risks. Interventions intended to provide direct diagnostic, therapeutic or preventive benefit for the individual child-subject must be justified by the expectation that they will be at least as advantageous to the individual child-subject, considering both risks and benefits, as any available alternative. Risks are to be justified in relation to anticipated benefits to the child.

The risk of interventions that are not intended to be of direct benefit to the child-subject must be justified in relation to anticipated benefits to society (generalizable knowledge). In general, the risk from such interventions should be minimal — that is, no more likely and not greater than the risk attached to routine medical or psychological examination of such children. When an ethical review committee is persuaded that the object of the research is sufficiently important, slight increases above minimal risk may be permitted.

Guideline 6: Research involving persons with mental or behavioural disorders

Before undertaking research involving individuals who by reason of mental or behavioural disorders are not capable of giving adequately informed consent, the investigator must ensure that:

— such persons will not be subjects of research that might equally well be carried out on persons in full possession of their mental faculties;

— the purpose of the research is to obtain knowledge relevant to the particular health needs of persons with mental or behavioural disorders;

— the consent of each subject has been obtained to the extent of that subject's capabilities, and a prospective subject's refusal to participate in non-clinical research is always respected;

— in the case of incompetent subjects, informed consent is obtained from the legal guardian or other duly authorized person;

— the degree of risk attached to interventions that are not intended to benefit the individual subject is low and commensurate with the importance of the knowledge to be gained; and

— interventions that are intended to provide therapeutic benefit are likely to be at least as advantageous to the individual subject as any alternative.

Commentary on Guideline 6

General considerations. Although the two populations differ in many respects, the ethical considerations discussed earlier in the case of children apply by and large to persons who are unable to give adequately informed consent by reason of mental or behavioural disorders. They should never be subjects of research that might equally well be carried out on adults in full possession of their mental faculties, but they are clearly the only subjects suitable for a large part of research into the origins and treatment of certain severe mental or behavioural disorders.

Consent of the individual. People with mental or behavioural disorders may not be capable of giving adequately informed consent. The willing cooperation of such prospective subjects should be sought to the extent that their mental state permits, and any objection on their part to taking part in any non-clinical research should always be respected. When an investigational intervention is intended to be of therapeutic benefit to a subject, the subject's objection should be respected unless there is no reasonable medical alternative and local law permits overriding the objection.

Proxy consent of the guardian. The Declaration of Helsinki states "In case of legal incompetence, informed consent should be obtained from the legal guardian in accordance with national legislation. Where physical or mental incapacity makes it impossible to obtain informed consent... permission from the responsible relative replaces that of the subject in accordance with national legislation" (Article I. 11).

The agreement of an immediate family member — whether spouse, parent, adult offspring or sibling — should be sought, but is sometimes of doubtful value, especially as families sometimes regard persons with mental or behavioural disorders as an unwelcome burden. In the case of an individual who has been committed to an institution by a court order, it may be necessary to seek legal authorization for involving the person in research.

Serious illness in persons who are unable to give adequately informed consent because of mental or behavioural disorders. Such persons who have, or are at risk of, serious illnesses such as HIV infection, cancer or hepatitis should not be deprived of the possible benefits of investigational drugs, vaccines or devices that show promise of therapeutic or preventive benefit, particularly when no superior or equivalent therapy or prevention is available. Their entitlement to access to such therapy or prevention is justified ethically on the same grounds as is such entitlement for other vulnerable groups (see Guideline 10). Persons who are unable to give adequately informed consent by reason of mental or behavioural disorders are, in general, not suitable subjects for formal clinical trials except those designed to be responsive to their particular health needs. Direct HIV infection of the brain may result in mental impairment; in the case of patients with such impairment, formal clinical trials of drugs, vaccines and other interventions designed to treat or prevent the impairment may be approved by an ethical review committee.

Anticipated incapacity to give informed consent. When it can be reasonably predicted that a competent person will lose the capacity to make valid decisions about medical care, as in the case of early manifestations of cognitive impairment due to HIV infection or Alzheimer's Disease, such a person may be asked to designate the conditions, if any, in which he or she would consent to becoming a research subject while unable to communicate, and to designate a person who will consent on his or her behalf in accordance with the subject's previously expressed wishes.

Guideline 7: Research involving prisoners

Prisoners with serious illness or at risk of serious illness should not arbitrarily be denied access to investigational drugs, vaccines or other agents that show promise of therapeutic or preventive benefit.

Commentary on Guideline 7

General considerations. Guideline 7 is not intended as an endorsement of involving prisoners as research subjects. The involvement of volunteer prisoners in biomedical research is permitted in very few countries, and even in those is controversial.

Advocates of allowing prisoners to participate in research argue that they are particularly suitable in that they are living in a standard physical and psychological environment; that unlike fully-employed or mobile populations they have time to participate in long-term experiments; and that they regard such participation as relief from the tedium of prison life, evidence of their social worth, and a chance to earn a small income.

Opponents claim that the consent of prisoners cannot be valid in that it is influenced by the hope of rewards and other expectations, such as earlier parole.

Although none of the international declarations bars prisoners from serving as subjects of biomedical research, the contradictory though persuasive arguments preclude an internationally agreed recommendation. However, where the practice is permitted, there should be provision for the independent monitoring of the research projects.

Prisoners and serious illness. Prisoners suffering from or at risk of serious illnesses such as HIV infection, cancer or hepatitis should not be deprived of the possible benefits of investigational drugs, vaccines or devices, particularly when no superior or equivalent products are available. Their entitlement to access to such therapy and prevention is justified ethically on the same grounds as is that of other vulnerable groups (see Guideline 10). However, as no diseases afflict prisoners only, one cannot sustain arguments analogous to those supporting the suitability of children and of persons with mental or behavioural disorders as subjects in formal clinical trials.

Guideline 8: Research involving subjects in underdeveloped communities

Before undertaking research involving subjects in underdeveloped communities, whether in developed or developing countries, the investigator must ensure that:

— **persons in underdeveloped communities will not ordinarily be involved in research that could be carried out reasonably well in developed communities;**
— **the research is responsive to the health needs and the priorities of the community in which it is to be carried out;**
— **every effort will be made to secure the ethical imperative that the consent of individual subjects be informed ; and**
— **the proposals for the research have been reviewed and approved by an ethical review committee that has among its members or consultants persons who are thoroughly familiar with the customs and traditions of the community.**

Commentary on Guideline 8

General considerations. Diseases that rarely or never occur in economically developed countries or communities exact a heavy toll of illness, disability or death in some communities that are socially and economically at risk of being exploited for research purposes. Research into the prevention and treatment of such diseases is needed and, in general, must be carried out in large part in the countries and communities at risk.

The ethical implications of research involving human subjects are identical in principle wherever the work is undertaken; they relate to respect for the dignity of each individual subject as well as to respect for communities, and protection of the rights and welfare of human subjects. Assessment of inherent risks is a pre-eminent concern. However, a number of subsidiary considerations apply particularly to research undertaken in underdeveloped communities of either developing or developed countries, by investigators and sponsors from developed countries or from developed institutions of developing countries.

Individuals and families in such communities are liable to exploitation for various reasons. Some of them may be relatively incapable of informed consent because they are illiterate, unfamiliar with the concepts of medicine held by the investigators, or living in communities in which the procedures typical of informed-consent discussions are unfamiliar or alien to the ethos of the community. Certain investigators may wish to take advantage of the lack in most developing countries of well-developed regulations or ethical review committees, which could have the effect of delaying access to research subjects; others may find it less expensive to conduct in developing countries research designed to develop drugs and other products for the markets of developed countries.

Guideline 8 is written on the presumption that research in developing countries or underdeveloped communities will generally be conducted by investigators and sponsored by agencies from developed countries or from developed communities of developing countries. Such investigators or sponsors may encounter practices that would be considered immoral in their own countries. This should be anticipated and the range of acceptable responses by the sponsors and investigators should be detailed in the protocol submitted to an ethical committee for review and approval.

Investigators must respect the ethical standards of their own countries and the cultural expectations of the societies in which research is undertaken, unless this implies a violation of a transcending moral rule. Investigators risk harming their reputation by pursuing work that host countries find acceptable but their own countries find offensive. Similarly, they may transgress the cultural values of the host countries by uncritically conforming to the expectations of their own.

Nature of the research. To guard against exploitation of individuals and families in socially and economically exploitable communities, sponsors and investigators who wish to conduct in such communities research that could be carried out reasonably well in developed communities must satisfy their national or local ethical review committees, and in the case of externally sponsored research the appropriate ethical review committee in the host country, that the research would not be exploitative. The reason for choosing an underdeveloped community should be made explicit.

The research conducted in underdeveloped communities should be responsive to the health needs and priorities of those communities. It should not exhaust resources which the community usually devotes to the health care of its members. If any product is to be developed, such as a new therapeutic agent, clear understanding should be reached among investigators, sponsors, representatives of the collaborating countries, and community leaders about what the community is to expect and what can or cannot be provided during and at the close of the research. Such understanding must be reached before the research is begun, to ensure that the research is truly responsive to the priorities of the community.

As a general rule, the sponsoring agency should ensure that, at the completion of successful testing, any product developed will be made reasonably available to inhabitants of the underdeveloped community in which the research was carried out; exceptions to this general requirement should be justified, and agreed to by all concerned parties before the research is begun.

Phase I drug studies and Phase I and II vaccine studies should be conducted only in developed communities of the country of the sponsor.

In general, Phase III vaccine trials and Phase II and III drug trials should be conducted simultaneously in the host community and the sponsoring country; they may be omitted in the sponsoring country on condition only that the drug or vaccine is designed to treat or prevent a disease or other condition that rarely or never occurs in the sponsoring country.

Informed consent. All reasonable efforts should be made to obtain the informed consent of each prospective subject according to the standards specified in Guidelines 1 to 3, to ensure that the rights of prospective subjects are respected. For example, when because of communication difficulties investigators cannot make prospective subjects sufficiently aware of the implications of participation to give adequately informed consent, the decision of each prospective subject on whether to consent should be elicited through a reliable intermediary such as a trusted community leader. In some cases other mechanisms, approved by an ethical review committee, may be more suitable. However consent is obtained, all prospective subjects must be clearly told that their participation is entirely voluntary, and that they are free to refuse to participate or to withdraw their participation at any time without loss of any entitlement. The investigator is required to ensure that each prospective subject is clearly told everything that would be conveyed if the study were to be conducted in a developed community and, further, to ensure that earnest attempts are made to enable the prospective subject to understand this information; otherwise, assurance of freedom to refuse or withdraw from participation would be meaningless.

All plans to use the above standard for informing, providing assistance with understanding, and assuring freedom to refuse or withdraw must be approved by an ethical review committee and supplemented with other means of assuring that the rights of prospective subjects are respected.

Ethical review. The ability to judge the ethical acceptability of various aspects of a research proposal requires a thorough understanding of a community's customs and traditions. The ethical review committee must have as either members or consultants persons with such understanding, so that the committee may evaluate proposed means of obtaining informed consent and otherwise respecting the rights of prospective subjects. Such persons should be able, for example, to identify appropriate members of the community to serve as intermediaries between investigators and subjects, to decide whether material benefits or inducements may be regarded as appropriate in the light of a community's gift-exchange traditions, and to provide safeguards for data and personal information that subjects consider to be private or sensitive.

HIV/AIDS considerations. HIV infection and AIDS are endemic in many of the world's countries and communities, both developed and developing. Some features of HIV/AIDS justify the involvement of people from underdeveloped communities in epidemiological research relevant to the HIV/AIDS pandemic as well as in research designed to test candidate drugs and vaccines for the treatment and prevention of HIV infection and AIDS. These include, but are not limited to, evidence that modes of transmission of the infection, and the natural history of the disease, may differ substantially among communities. Moreover, strains of HIV are different in various regions of the world, and the current scientific understanding is that different strains may respond differently to vaccines or drugs. If research were conducted only in developed countries and communities, developing countries could be deprived of many of the benefits of such research. Therefore, participation in HIV/AIDS research of inhabitants of appropriately selected underdeveloped communities should be encouraged, provided their rights and welfare are adequately safeguarded as set forth in Guideline 8.

Guideline 9: Informed consent in epidemiological studies

For several types of epidemiological research individual informed consent is either impracticable or inadvisable. In such cases the ethical review committee should determine whether it is ethically acceptable to proceed without individual informed consent and whether the investigator's plans to protect the safety and respect the privacy of research subjects and to maintain the confidentiality of the data are adequate.

Commentary on Guideline 9

General considerations. For epidemiological studies it is normal for investigators to secure the agreement and cooperation of the national or local authority responsible for public health in the population to be studied. In the case of a community in which collective decision-making is customary it is also advisable to seek the agreement of the community, usually through its chosen representatives.

Informed consent. Epidemiological studies that require the examination of documents, such as medical records, or of anonymous "leftover" samples of blood, urine, saliva or tissue specimens may be conducted without the consent of the individuals concerned, as long as their right to confidentiality is assured by the study methods.

When the focus of a study is an entire community rather than individual human subjects — for example, to test the use of an additive in a community's water supply, or a new health care procedure or method, or a new method of control of disease vectors such as mosquitoes or rats — individual consent or an individual's refusal to be exposed to the intervention would be meaningless unless the individual were willing to leave the community. However, individuals may refuse to submit to such procedures as questionnaires or blood tests designed to obtain data for evaluating the intervention.

When epidemiological studies entail personal contact between investigators and individual subjects, the general requirements for informed consent are directly applicable. When they involve individuals primarily as members of population groups, it may be acceptable not to obtain the informed consent of each individual. In the case of population groups with social structures, common customs, and an acknowledged leadership, the investigator will need to secure the cooperation and obtain the agreement of the group's leadership. In the case of groups defined solely in demographic or statistical terms, with neither leaders nor representatives, the investigator must satisfy an ethical review committee that the safety of the research subjects and the confidentiality of the data will be strictly safeguarded.

Consent is not required for the use of publicly available information, but the investigator should know that countries and communities differ with regard to what information about individuals is considered public. Investigators who use such information should avoid disclosure of personally sensitive information.

In the case of studies of certain forms of social behaviour, an ethical review committee may determine that it would be inadvisable to seek individual informed consent because to do so would frustrate the purpose of a study; for example, prospective subjects on being informed of the behaviour to be studied would change the behaviour. The review committee must be satisfied that there will be adequate safeguards of confidentiality and that the importance of the objectives of the research is in proportion to the risks to the subjects.

Investigators who propose to carry out epidemiological studies should consult *International Guidelines for Ethical Review of Epidemiological Studies* (CIOMS, 1991).

Selection of Research Subjects

Guideline 10: Equitable distribution of burdens and benefits

Individuals or communities to be invited to be subjects of research should be selected in such a way that the burdens and benefits of the research will be equitably distributed. Special justification is required for inviting vulnerable individuals and, if they are selected, the means of protecting their rights and welfare must be particularly strictly applied.

Commentary on Guideline 10

General considerations. In general, the equitable distribution of the burdens and the benefits of participation in research raises no serious problems when the intended subjects do not include vulnerable individuals or communities. Occasionally, when research is designed to evaluate therapeutic agents widely perceived to offer substantial advantages over those generally available, it may be appropriate to publicize widely the opportunity to participate in the research or to establish outreach programmes for individuals or groups who have no ready access to information about research programmes.

Equitable distribution of the burdens and benefits of research participation is generally more difficult when the intended subjects include vulnerable individuals or groups. Classes of individuals traditionally considered vulnerable are those with limited capacity or freedom to consent. They are the subject of specific guidelines in this document and include children, persons who because of mental or behavioural disorders are incapable of giving informed consent, and prisoners. Ethical justification of their involvement usually requires that investigators satisfy ethical review committees that:

— the research could not be carried out reasonably well with less vulnerable subjects;
— the research is intended to obtain knowledge that will lead to improved diagnosis, prevention or treatment of diseases or other health problems characteristic of or unique to the vulnerable class, either the actual subjects or other similarly situated members of the vulnerable class;
— research subjects and other members of the vulnerable class from which subjects are recruited will ordinarily be assured reasonable access to any diagnostic, preventive or therapeutic products that will become available as a consequence of the research;
— the risks attached to research that is not intended to benefit individual subjects will be minimal, unless an ethical review committee authorizes a slight increase above minimal risk (see Guideline 5); and
— when the prospective subjects are either incompetent or otherwise substantially unable to give informed consent, their agreement will be supplemented by the proxy consent of their legal guardians or other duly authorized representatives.

Other vulnerable social groups. The quality of the consent of prospective subjects who are junior or subordinate members of a hierarchical group requires careful consideration, as their agreement to volunteer may be unduly influenced by the expectation, whether justified or not, of preferential treatment or by fear of disapproval or retaliation if they refuse. Examples of such groups are medical and nursing students, subordinate hospital and laboratory personnel, employees of pharmaceutical companies, and members of the armed forces or police.

Because they work in close proximity to investigators or disciplinary superiors, they tend to be called upon more often than others to serve as research subjects, and this could result in inequitable distribution of the burdens and benefits of research.

Other groups or classes may also be considered vulnerable. They include residents of nursing homes, people receiving welfare benefits or social assistance and other poor people and the unemployed, patients in emergency rooms, some ethnic and racial minority groups, homeless persons, nomads, refugees, and patients with incurable disease. To the extent that these and other classes of people have attributes resembling those of classes identified as vulnerable, the need for special protection of their rights and welfare should be considered.

Persons with HIV infection or at risk of contracting HIV infection. Persons in this category are not vulnerable in the sense of having limited capacity to consent. However, certain features of HIV infection and of the AIDS pandemic have prompted reconsideration of some aspects of the ethics of research involving human subjects; as a result, various countries have developed policies and practices designed to be responsive to the special problems presented by HIV infection; some of these problems are incorporated in the following paragraphs. Although this commentary concerns problems associated with HIV infection, the basic principles apply equally to problems associated with other more or less similar conditions.

Drugs and other therapies that have not yet been licensed for general availability because studies designed to establish their safety and efficacy remain to be completed are sometimes made available to persons with HIV infection. This is compatible with the Declaration of Helsinki, Article II.1, which states "...the physician must be free to use a new diagnostic or therapeutic measure, if in his or her judgment it offers hope of saving life, reestablishing health or alleviating suffering."

Drugs and other therapies that are made available, because they show promise of therapeutic benefit, to persons not considered vulnerable should be made equally available to members of vulnerable populations, particularly when no superior or equivalent approaches to therapy are available; children, pregnant or nursing women, persons with mental disorders who are not capable of giving informed consent, and prisoners are entitled to equal access to the benefits of such investigational agents unless there is good reason, such as a medical contraindication, not to afford such access.

When women take investigational drugs for HIV infection, special precautions are often needed. Women who are not pregnant when they begin to take such drugs should be counselled about reliable contraception. In developed countries, nursing mothers who ask to be treated with investigational drugs for HIV infection should be advised that they must discontinue breast-feeding while taking such drugs, unless there is clear evidence that the drug does not appear in milk. In each case in which an investigational drug is administered to a pregnant or nursing woman, there should be careful monitoring and reporting of the effects, if any, on the fetus or child.

31

Although it is generally required that research be conducted on less vulnerable populations before involving more vulnerable populations, some exceptions are justified. In general, children are not suitable subjects for Phase I drug trials or for Phase I or II vaccine trials, but in some cases such trials may be permissible after clinical trials in adults have shown some degree of therapeutic effect. For example, a Phase II vaccine trial seeking evidence of immunogenicity in infants may be justified in the case of a vaccine that has shown evidence of preventing or slowing progression from asymptomatic HIV infection to disease in adults. Additional examples are provided in the commentaries on Guidelines 6 and 8.

The life-threatening and infectious nature of HIV/AIDS does not justify any suspension of the rights of research subjects to informed consent, voluntary participation in or withdrawal from the study, or protection of confidentiality. In the case of research protocols that provide for diagnostic tests for HIV infection, the procedures for obtaining informed consent should be supplemented by counselling in which each subject is informed about AIDS and HIV infection, advised to avoid risky behaviour, and advised of the risk of social discrimination against individuals who are thought to be HIV-infected or at risk of such infection. In the case of patients with HIV disease or persons becoming aware of being HIV-infected, research teams should provide them with necessary services or refer them for follow-up.

Participation in drug and vaccine trials in the field of HIV infection and AIDS may impose on the research subjects significant associated risks of social discrimination or harm; such risks merit consideration equal to that given to the adverse medical consequences of the drugs and vaccines. Efforts must be made to reduce their likelihood and severity. For example, participants in vaccine trials must be enabled to demonstrate that their HIV seropositivity is due to their having been vaccinated rather than to natural infection. This may be accomplished by providing subjects with documents attesting to their participation in vaccine trials, or by maintaining a confidential register of trial participants, from which information can be made available to outside agencies at a participant's request.

Guideline 11: Selection of pregnant or nursing (breastfeeding) women as research subjects

Pregnant or nursing women should in no circumstances be the subjects of non-clinical research unless the research carries no more than minimal risk to the fetus or nursing infant and the object of the research is to obtain new knowledge about pregnancy or lactation. As a general rule, pregnant or nursing women should not be subjects of any clinical trials except such trials as are designed to protect or advance the health of pregnant or nursing women or fetuses or nursing infants, and for which women who are not pregnant or nursing would not be suitable subjects.

Commentary on Guideline 11

General considerations. In general, pregnant and nursing women are not suitable subjects of formal clinical trials other than those designed to respond to the health needs of such women or their fetuses or nursing infants. Examples of such trials would be a trial designed to test the safety and efficacy of a drug for reducing perinatal transmission of HIV infection from mother to child, a trial of a device for detecting fetal abnormalities, or trials of therapies for conditions associated with or aggravated by pregnancy, such as nausea and vomiting, hypertension or diabetes. The justification for their participation in such clinical trials would be that they should not be deprived arbitrarily of the opportunity to benefit from investigational drugs, vaccines or other agents that promise therapeutic or preventive benefit. In all cases risks to women subjects, fetuses and infants should be minimized, as far as sound research design permits.

A woman may decide to discontinue nursing to become eligible to participate in clinical research, but this is not to be encouraged, particularly in developing countries, where cessation of breast-feeding may be harmful to the nursing child and also increase the risk of another pregnancy.

Selection of women as research subjects. Women in most societies have been discriminated against with regard to their involvement in research. Women who are biologically capable of becoming pregnant have been customarily excluded from formal clinical trials of drugs, vaccines, and devices owing to concern about undetermined risks to the fetus. Consequently, relatively little is known about the safety and efficacy of most drugs, vaccines, or devices for such women, and this lack of knowledge can be dangerous. For example, Thalidomide caused much more extensive damage than it would have if its first administration to such women had been in the context of a formal, carefully-monitored clinical trial.

A general policy of excluding from such clinical trials women biologically capable of becoming pregnant is unjust in that it deprives women as a class of persons of the benefits of the new knowledge derived from the trials. Further, it is an affront to their right of self-determination. The exclusion of such women can be justified only on such grounds as evidence or suspicion that a particular drug or vaccine is mutagenic or teratogenic. Nevertheless, although women of child-bearing age should be given the opportunity to participate in research, they should be helped to understand that the research could include risks to the fetus.

Premenopausal women have also been excluded from participation in many research activities, including non-clinical studies, that do not entail administration of drugs or vaccines, in case the physiological changes associated with various phases of the menstrual cycle would complicate interpretation of research data. Consequently, much less is known of women's than of men's normal physiological processes. This, too, is unjust in that it deprives women as a class of persons of the benefits of such knowledge.

Informed consent. Obtaining the informed consent of women, including those who are pregnant or nursing, usually presents no special problems. In some cultures, however, women's rights to exercise self-determination and thus give valid informed consent are not acknowledged. In such cases, women should not normally be involved in research for which societies that recognize these rights require informed consent. Nevertheless, women who have serious illnesses or who are at risk of developing such illnesses should not be deprived of opportunities to receive investigational therapies when there are no better alternatives, even though they may not consent for themselves. Efforts must be made to let such women know of these opportunities and to invite them to decide whether they wish to accept the investigational therapy, even though the formal consent must be obtained from another person, usually a man. Such invitations may best be extended by women who understand the culture sufficiently well to discern whether prospective recipients of investigational therapies genuinely wish to accept or reject the therapy.

Research related to termination of pregnancy. No recommendation is made regarding the acceptability of research relating to the termination of pregnancy, or undertaken in anticipation of termination of pregnancy. The acceptability of such research depends on religious belief, cultural traditions and national legislation.

Confidentiality of Data

Guideline 12: Safeguarding confidentiality

The investigator must establish secure safeguards of the confidentiality of research data. Subjects should be told of the limits to the investigators' ability to safeguard confidentiality and of the anticipated consequences of breaches of confidentiality.

Commentary on Guideline 12

General considerations. The Declaration of Helsinki, Article I.6, states: "The right of the research subject to safeguard his or her integrity must always be respected. Every precaution should be taken to respect the privacy of the subject and to minimize the impact of the study on the subject's physical and mental integrity and on the personality of the subject." The customary approach to showing respect for privacy is by obtaining prior informed consent to releases of research data and minimizing the possibility of a breach of confidentiality. If the requirement of individual informed consent is to be waived by an ethical review committee, alternative measures should be taken. Such measures are discussed in *International Guidelines for Ethical Review of Epidemiological Studies* (CIOMS, 1991).

Confidentiality between physician and patient. Patients in therapeutic relationships with their physicians have the right to expect that all information will be held in strict confidence and disclosed only to those who need, or have a legal right to, the information, such as nurses and technicians, to treat the patients. A treating physician should not disclose any identifying data about patients to an investigator unless the patients have first given their consent to such disclosure.

Physicians and other health care professionals record the details of their observations and interventions in medical and other records. Epidemiologists and other investigators often make use of such records. In studies of medical records it is usually impracticable to obtain the informed consent of each identifiable patient. Accordingly, an ethical review committee may waive the requirement for informed consent. In institutions in which records may be used for research purposes without the informed consent of identifiable patients, it is advisable to notify patients generally of such practices; notification is usually by means of a statement in patient-information brochures.

In the case of research limited to subjects' medical records, access must be approved by an ethical review committee and must be supervised by a person who is fully aware of the confidentiality requirements.

Confidentiality between investigator and subject. Research relating to individuals and groups may involve the collection and storage of data that, if disclosed to third parties, could cause harm or distress. Investigators should arrange to protect the confidentiality of such data by, for example, omitting information that might lead to the identification of individual subjects, limiting access to the data, or other means.

Prospective subjects should be informed of limits to the investigators' ability to ensure strict confidentiality and of the foreseeable adverse social consequences of limitations or breaches of confidentiality. In some cases investigators are required to communicate data from records to a national drug registration authority or to an industrial sponsor of the research. Some jurisdictions require the reporting of, for instance, certain communicable diseases to public health authorities or evidence of child abuse or neglect to appropriate agencies. These and similar limits to the ability to maintain confidentiality should be anticipated and disclosed to prospective subjects.

Compensation of Research Subjects for Accidental Injury

Guideline 13: Right of subjects to compensation

Research subjects who suffer physical injury as a result of their participation are entitled to such financial or other assistance as would compensate them equitably for any temporary or permanent impairment or disability. In the case of death, their dependants are entitled to material compensation. The right to compensation may not be waived.

Commentary on Guideline 13

Accidental injury. Accidental injury due to procedures performed exclusively to accomplish the purposes of research rarely results in death or in permanent or temporary impairment or disability. Death, impairment or disability is much more likely to result from investigational diagnostic, preventive or therapeutic interventions. In general, however, death or serious injury is less likely to result from investigational therapies administered in the context of properly designed, conducted and sanctioned studies than from similar standard therapies in routine medical practice. Usually, human research subjects are in exceptionally favourable circumstances in that they are under close and continuing observation by qualified investigators alert to detecting the earliest signs of untoward reactions. Such favourable conditions are less likely in medical practice.

Equitable compensation. Compensation is owed to subjects who sustain significant physical injury from procedures performed solely to accomplish the purposes of research. Justice requires that every subject of biomedical research be automatically entitled to fair compensation for any such injury. Compensation is generally not owed to research subjects who suffer expected or foreseen adverse reactions from investigational therapies or other procedures performed to diagnose or prevent disease. Such reactions are not different in kind from those that occur in medical practice.

When, as in the early stages of drug testing, it is unclear whether a procedure is performed primarily for research or for therapeutic purposes, the ethical review committee should determine in advance the injuries for which subjects will be compensated and those for which they will not; prospective subjects should be informed of the review committee's decisions, as part of the informed consent process.

Subjects should not be required to waive their rights to compensation or to show negligence or lack of a reasonable degree of skill on the part of the investigator in order to claim compensation. The informed consent process or form should contain no words that would absolve an investigator from responsibility in the case of accidental injury, or that would imply that subjects would waive their legal rights, including the right to seek compensation for injury.

In some societies the right to compensation for accidental injury is not acknowledged. Therefore, when giving their informed consent to participate, research subjects should be told whether there is provision for compensation in case of physical injury, and the circumstances in which they or their dependants would receive it.

Obligation of the sponsor to pay. The sponsor, whether a pharmaceutical company, a government, or an institution, should agree, before the research begins, to provide compensation for any physical injury for which subjects are entitled to compensation. Sponsors are advised to obtain adequate insurance against risks to cover compensation, independent of proof of fault.

Review Procedures

Guideline 14: Constitution and responsibilities of ethical review committees

All proposals to conduct research involving human subjects must be submitted for review and approval to one or more independent ethical and scientific review committees. The investigator must obtain such approval of the proposal to conduct research before the research is begun.

Commentary on Guideline 14

General considerations. The provisions for review of research involving human subjects are influenced by political institutions, the organization of medical practice and research, and the degree of autonomy accorded to medical investigators. Whatever the circumstances, however, society has a dual responsibility to ensure that:

- all drugs, devices and vaccines under investigation in human subjects meet adequate standards of safety; and
- the provisions of the Declaration of Helsinki are applied in all biomedical research involving human subjects.

Assessment of safety. Authority to assess the safety and quality of medicines and vaccines intended for use in humans is most effectively vested in a multidisciplinary advisory committee. In many cases such committees will function best if they operate at the national level; in other instances they are most effective at regional or local level. Clinicians, clinical pharmacologists, pharmacologists, microbiologists, epidemiologists, statisticians and other experts have important contributions to offer to such assessment. Many countries lack the resources to assess technical data independently according to procedures and standards now required in the more developed countries. Improvement in this respect depends, in the short term, on more efficient exchange of information internationally.

Ethical review committees. Scientific review and ethical review cannot be clearly separated: scientifically unsound research on human subjects is *ipso facto* unethical in that it may expose subjects to risk or inconvenience to no purpose. Normally, therefore, ethical review committees consider both the scientific and the ethical aspects of proposed research.

Scientific review. The Declaration of Helsinki, Article I.1, states that "biomedical research involving human subjects must conform to generally accepted scientific principles and should be based on adequately performed laboratory and animal experimentation and on a thorough knowledge of the scientific literature."

Committees competent to review and approve scientific aspects of clinical trials must be multidisciplinary, much like those specified earlier for assessment of safety. In many cases such committees operate most effectively at the national level. A national scientific review committee offers several advantages over local committees. First, consolidating the necessary expertise in one group allows members to deepen their knowledge in the field, thereby improving the quality and utility of the review. Second, a national committee's awareness of all proposals for research in the country facilitates the performance of another essential function, the selection of those protocols most likely to achieve the nation's health research objectives.

If an ethical review committee considers a research proposal scientifically sound, or verifies that a competent expert body has found it so, it will then consider whether any known or possible risks to the subjects are justified by the expected benefits (and whether the methods of carrying out the research will minimize harm and maximize benefit) and, if so, whether the procedures proposed for obtaining informed consent are satisfactory and those proposed for selection of subjects are equitable.

Risks and benefits. The Declaration of Helsinki forbids the imposition of unwarranted risks on human research subjects. Article I.4 requires that "the importance of the objective is in proportion to the inherent risk to the subject." The need for means of preventing or treating HIV infection or AIDS, for example, is obvious justification of research aimed at developing such treatment or prevention. However, it may not be possible to justify clinical testing of all investigational substances. Clinical testing must be preceded by sufficient laboratory experiments, including, when appropriate, animal testing, to demonstrate a reasonable probability of success without undue risk. Such preliminary testing is implied by the Declaration of Helsinki, Article I.7, which requires forgoing research involving human subjects unless "the hazards involved are believed to be predictable", and by Article I.5, which requires that clinical testing "be preceded by careful assessment of predictable risks in comparison with foreseeable benefits to the subject or to others."

Ideally, when benefits are intended for society but not for the subject, the subjects should be individuals who are fully capable of informed consent and who understand and accept the risks. Thus, unless there is specially strong justification, Phases I and II of vaccine testing and Phase I of drug testing should not involve subjects with limited capacity to consent or who are otherwise vulnerable. The requirement of the Declaration of Helsinki, Article III.2, that "subjects should be volunteers—either healthy persons or patients for whom the experimental design is not related to the patient's illness" is not to be disregarded lightly.

In Phases II and III of drug testing and Phase III of vaccine testing, when benefits are intended for the subjects and they are reasonably likely to be realized, it is permissible to involve members of vulnerable groups and persons with limited capacity to consent. However, as required by the Declaration of Helsinki, Article II.3, "every patient — including those of a control group, if any — should be assured of the best proven diagnostic and therapeutic method." Therefore, if there is already an approved and accepted drug for the condition that a candidate drug is designed to treat, placebo for controls usually cannot be justified.

Ethical justification to begin a randomized clinical trial also meets the requirements of Article II.3. The therapies (or other interventions) to be compared must be regarded as equally advantageous to the prospective subjects: there should be no scientific evidence to establish the superiority of one over another. Moreover, no other intervention must be known to be superior to those being compared in the clinical trial, unless eligibility to participate is limited to persons who have been unsuccessfully treated with the other superior intervention or to persons who are aware of the other intervention and its superiority and have chosen not to accept it.

For each randomized clinical trial there should be a data and safety monitoring committee, responsible for monitoring the data obtained in the course of a study and for making recommendations to the sponsors and investigators about modifying or terminating the study, or about amending the informed-consent process or form. Such recommendations are made in response to the committee's detection of adverse events of which the nature, frequency or magnitude had not been anticipated by the investigators or sponsors as they planned the study, or of evidence that one of the therapies or preventive measures being tested in the clinical trial is superior to another. During the planning stage of a clinical trial, stopping-rules should be established to guide the data and safety monitoring committee in determining when it should recommend termination of the study.

National or local review. Review committees may be created under the aegis of national or local health administrations, national medical research councils or other nationally-representative bodies. In a highly centralized administration, a national review committee may be constituted for both the scientific and the ethical review of research protocols. In countries where medical research is not centrally directed, protocols are more effectively and conveniently reviewed from the ethical standpoint at a local or regional level. The competence of a local committee may be confined exclusively to a single research institution or may extend to all human-subject biomedical research undertaken within a defined geographical area. The basic responsibilities of local ethical review committees are twofold:
- to verify that all proposed interventions, and particularly the administration of drugs and vaccines or use of medical devices under development, have been assessed by a competent expert body as acceptably safe to be undertaken in human subjects; and
- to ensure that all other ethical concerns arising from a protocol are satisfactorily resolved both in principle and in practice.

Committee membership. Local review committees should be so composed as to be able to provide complete and adequate review of the research activities referred to them. They should include physicians, scientists and other professionals, such as nurses, lawyers, ethicists and clergy, as well as lay persons qualified to represent the cultural and moral values of the community. The membership should include both men and women. Committees that often review research directed at specific diseases or impairments, such as AIDS or paraplegia, should consider the advantages of including as members or consultants patients with such diseases or impairments. Similarly, committees that review research involving such vulnerable groups as children, students, aged persons or employees should consider the advantages of including representatives of, or advocates for, such groups. Membership should be rotated periodically with the aim of blending the advantages of experience with those of openness to cultural and scientific evolution. Independence from the investigators and avoidance of conflict of interest are maintained by excluding from the assessment of a proposal any member with a direct interest in the proposal.

Need for particularly stringent review requirements. The requirements of review committees should be particularly stringent in the case of proposed research involving children, pregnant and nursing women, persons with mental or behavioural disorders, communities unfamiliar with modern clinical concepts, and other vulnerable social groups, and in the case of invasive non-clinical research. In considering such proposals the review committee should be especially attentive in determining that selection of research subjects is both equitable (designed to distribute fairly the burdens and benefits of research) and likely to minimize risk to subjects.

Multicentre research. Some research projects are designed to be conducted in a number of sites in different communities or countries. Generally, to ensure that the results will be valid, the study must be conducted in an identical way at each of the different sites. Such studies include multicentre clinical trials, evaluation of health service programmes, and various kinds of epidemiological research. In such studies local ethical review committees must either accept or reject the protocol in its entirety; they must not impose requirements to change doses of drugs, to change inclusion or exclusion criteria, or to make other similar modifications. In some such studies, scientific and ethical review may be facilitated by agreement among institutions to accept the results of review by a single review committee, whose members would include representatives of ethical review committees at each of the places in which the research is to be conducted.

Sanctions. Ethical review committees generally have no authority to impose sanctions on investigators who violate ethical standards in the conduct of research involving human subjects. However, they should be required to report to institutional or governmental authorities any serious or continuing noncompliance with ethical standards as they are reflected in protocols that they have approved. Failure to submit a protocol to the committee should be considered a violation of ethical standards.

Sanctions imposed by institutional, governmental, professional or other authorities possessing disciplinary power should be employed as a last resort. Preferred methods of control include cultivation of an atmosphere of mutual trust, and education and support to promote in investigators and in sponsors the capacity for ethical conduct of research.

41

Should sanctions become necessary, they should be directed at the noncompliant investigators or sponsors. They may include fines or suspension of eligibility to receive research funding, to use investigational therapies, or to practise medicine. Refusal to publish the results of research conducted unethically, as prescribed in the Declaration of Helsinki, Article I.8, may be considered, as may refusal to accept unethically obtained data submitted in support of an application for drug registration. However, these sanctions deprive of benefit not only the errant investigator or sponsor but also that segment of society intended to benefit from the research; such possible consequences merit careful consideration.

Publications of reports of the results of research involving human subjects should include, when appropriate, a statement that the research was conducted in accordance with these guidelines. Departures, if any, from these guidelines should be explained and justified in the report submitted for publication.

Information to be provided by investigators. Whatever the procedure adopted for ethical review, such review should be based on a detailed protocol comprising:
— a clear statement of the research objectives, having regard to the present state of knowledge, and a justification for undertaking the investigation in human subjects;
— a precise description of all proposed interventions, including intended dosages of drugs and planned duration of treatment;
— a description of plans to withdraw or withhold standard therapies in the course of the research;
— a description of the plans for statistical analysis of the study, which includes a calculation of the statistical power of the study, specifies the criteria for terminating the study, and demonstrates that the proper number of subjects will be recruited;
— the criteria determining admission and withdrawal of individual subjects, including full details of the procedure for seeking and obtaining informed consent;
— an account of any economic or other inducements to participate, such as offers of cash payments, gifts, or free services or facilities, and of any financial obligations assumed by the subjects, such as payment for medical services; and
— for research carrying more than minimal risk of physical injury, an account of plans, if any, to provide medical therapy for such injury and to provide compensation for research-related disability or death.
Information should also be included to establish:
— the safety of each proposed intervention and of any drug or vaccine to be tested, including the results of relevant laboratory and animal research;
— the anticipated benefits and the risks of participation;

- the means proposed to obtain individual informed consent or, when a prospective subject is not capable of informed consent, satisfactory assurance that proxy consent will be obtained from a duly authorized person and that the rights and welfare of each subject will be adequately protected;
- the identification of the organization that is sponsoring the research and a detailed account of the sponsor's financial commitments to the research institution, investigators, research subjects and, when appropriate, the community;
- plans to inform subjects about harms and benefits during the study, and of the results of the study at its conclusion;
- an explanation of who will be involved in the research, their age, sex and circumstances, and, if any classes are excluded, the justification for the exclusion;
- justification for involving as research subjects persons with limited capacity to consent or members of vulnerable social groups;
- evidence that the investigator is qualified and experienced and is assured of adequate facilities for the safe and efficient conduct of the research;
- provisions that will be made for protecting the confidentiality of data; and,
- the nature of any other ethical considerations involved, together with an indication that the principles of the Declaration of Helsinki will be implemented.

Externally Sponsored Research

Guideline 15: Obligations of sponsoring and host countries

Externally sponsored research entails two ethical obligations:
- **An external sponsoring agency should submit the research protocol to ethical and scientific review according to the standards of the country of the sponsoring agency, and the ethical standards applied should be no less exacting than they would be in the case of research carried out in that country.**
- **After scientific and ethical approval in the country of the sponsoring agency, the appropriate authorities of the host country, including a national or local ethical review committee or its equivalent, should satisfy themselves that the proposed research meets their own ethical requirements.**

Commentary on Guideline 15

Definition. The term "externally sponsored research" refers to research undertaken in a host country but sponsored, financed, and sometimes wholly or partly carried out by an external international or national

43

agency, with the collaboration or agreement of the appropriate authorities, institutions and personnel of the host country.

Ethical and scientific review. Committees in both the country of the sponsoring agency and the host country have responsibility for conducting both scientific and ethical review, as well as the authority to withhold approval of research proposals that fail to meet their scientific or ethical standards. Special responsibilites may be assigned to review committees in the two countries when a sponsor or investigator in a developed country proposes to carry out research in a developing country. When the external sponsor is an international agency the research protocol must be reviewed according to its own independent ethical review procedures and standards.

Committees in the external sponsoring country or international agency have a special responsibility to determine whether the scientific methods are sound and suitable for the aims of the research, whether the drugs, vaccines or devices to be studied meet adequate standards of safety, whether there is sound justification for conducting the research in the host country rather than in the country of the external sponsoring agency, and that the proposed research does not in principle violate the ethical standards of the external sponsoring country or international organization.

Committees in the host country have the special responsibility to determine whether the goals of the research are responsive to the health needs and priorities of the host country. Moreover, because of their better understanding of the culture in which the research is proposed to be carried out, they have special responsibility for assuring the equitable selection of subjects and the acceptability of plans to obtain informed consent, to respect privacy, to maintain confidentiality, and to offer benefits that will not be considered excessive inducements to consent.

In short, ethical review in the external sponsoring country may be limited to ensuring compliance with broadly stated ethical standards, on the understanding that ethical review committees in the host country will have greater competence in reviewing the detailed plans for compliance in view of their better understanding of the cultural and moral values of the population in which the research is proposed to be conducted.

Research designed to develop therapeutic, diagnostic or preventive products. When externally sponsored research is initiated and financed by an industrial sponsor such as a pharmaceutical company, it is in the interest of the host country to require that the research proposal be submitted with the comments of a responsible authority of the initiating country, such as a health administration, research council, or academy of medicine or science.

Externally sponsored research designed to develop a therapeutic, diagnostic or preventive product must be responsive to the health needs of the host country. It should be conducted only in host countries in which the disease or other condition for which the product is indicated is an important problem. As a general rule, the sponsoring agency should agree in advance of the research that any product developed though such research will be made reasonably available to the inhabitants of the host community or country at the completion of successful testing. Exceptions to this general requirement should be justified and agreed to by all concerned parties before the research begins. Consideration should be given to whether the sponsoring agency should agree to maintain in the host country, after the research has been completed, health services and facilities established for purposes of the study.

Obligations of external sponsors. An important secondary objective of externally sponsored collaborative research is to help develop the host country's capacity to carry out similar research projects independently, including their ethical review. Accordingly, external sponsors are expected to employ and, if necessary, train local individuals to function as investigators, research assistants, data managers or in other similar capacities. When indicated, sponsors should also provide facilities and personnel to make necessary health-care services available to the population from which research subjects are recruited. Although sponsors are not obliged to provide health-care facilities or personnel beyond that which is necessary for the conduct of the research, to do so is morally praiseworthy. However, sponsors have an obligation to ensure that subjects who suffer injury as a consequence of research interventions obtain medical treatment free of charge, and that compensation is provided for death or disability occurring as a consequence of such injury (see Guideline 13 for a statement of the scope and limits of such obligations). Also, sponsors and investigators should refer for health care services subjects or prospective subjects who are found to have diseases unrelated to the research, and should advise prospective subjects who are rejected as research subjects because they do not meet health criteria for admission to the investigation to seek medical care. Sponsors are expected to ensure that research subjects and the communities from which they are recruited are not made worse off as a result of the research (apart from justifiable risks of research interventions) — for example, by the diversion of scarce local resources to research activities. Sponsors may disclose to the proper authorities in the host country information that relates to the health of the country or community, discovered in the course of a study.

External sponsors are expected to provide, as necessary, reasonable amounts of financial, educational and other assistance to enable the host country to develop its own capacity for independent ethical review of research proposals and to form independent and competent scientific and ethical review committees. To avoid conflict of interest, and to assure the independence of committees, such assistance should not be provided directly to the committees; rather funds should be made available to the host-country government or to the host research-institution.

Obligations of sponsors will vary with the circumstances of particular studies and the needs of host countries. The sponsors' obligations in particular studies should be clarified before research is begun. The research protocol should specify what, if any, resources, facilities, assistance and other goods or services will be made available, during and after the research, to the community from which the subjects are drawn and to the host country. The details of these arrangements should be agreed by the sponsor, officials of the host country, other interested parties, and, when relevant, the community from which subjects are to be drawn. The ethical review committee in the host country should determine whether any or all of these details should be made a part of the consent process.

Annex 1

WORLD MEDICAL ASSOCIATION DECLARATION OF HELSINKI

Recommendations guiding physicians
in biomedical research involving human subjects

Adopted by the 18th World Medical Assembly
Helsinki, Finland, June 1964

and amended by the
29th World Medical Assembly
Tokyo, Japan, October 1975
35th World Medical Assembly
Venice, Italy, October 1983
and the
41st World Medical Assembly
Hong Kong, September 1989

INTRODUCTION

It is the mission of the physician to safeguard the health of the people. His or her knowledge and conscience are dedicated to the fulfillment of this mission.

The Declaration of Geneva of the World Medical Association binds the physician with the words, "The health of my patient will be my first consideration," and the International Code of Medical Ethics declares that, "A physician shall act only in the patient's interest when providing medical care which might have the effect of weakening the physical and mental condition of the patient."

The purpose of biomedical research involving human subjects must be to improve diagnostic, therapeutic and prophylactic procedures and the understanding of the aetiology and pathogenesis of disease.

In current medical practice most diagnostic, therapeutic or prophylactic procedures involve hazards. This applies especially to biomedical research.

Medical progress is based on research which ultimately must rest in part on experimentation involving human subjects.

In the field of biomedical research a fundamental distinction must be recognized between medical research in which the aim is essentially diagnostic or therapeutic for a patient, and medical research, the essential object of which is purely scientific and without implying direct diagnostic or therapeutic value to the person subjected to the research.

Special caution must be exercised in the conduct of research which may affect the environment, and the welfare of animals used for research must be respected.

Because it is essential that the results of laboratory experiments be applied to human beings to further scientific knowledge and to help suffering humanity, the World Medical Association has prepared the following recommendations as a guide to every physician in biomedical research involving human subjects. They should be kept under review in the future. It must be stressed that the standards as drafted are only a guide to physicians all over the world. Physicians are not relieved from criminal, civil and ethical responsibilities under the laws of their own countries.

I. BASIC PRINCIPLES

1. Biomedical research involving human subjects must conform to generally accepted scientific principles and should be based on adequately performed laboratory and animal experimentation and a thorough knowledge of the scientific literature.

2. The design and performance of each experimental procedure involving human subjects should be clearly formulated in an experimental protocol which should be transmitted for consideration, comment and guidance to a specially appointed committee independent of the investigator and the sponsor, provided that this independent committee is in conformity with the laws and regulations of the country in which the research experiment is performed.

3. Biomedical research involving human subjects should be conducted only by scientifically qualified persons and under the supervision of a clinically competent medical person. The responsibility for the human subject must always rest with a medically qualified person and never rest on the subject of the research, even though the subject has given his or her consent.

4. Biomedical research involving human subjects cannot legitimately be carried out unless the importance of the objective is in proportion to the inherent risk to the subject.

5. Every biomedical research project involving human subjects should be preceded by careful assessment of predictable risks in comparison with foreseeable benefits to the subject or to others. Concern for the interests of the subject must always prevail over the interests of science and society.

6. The right of the research subject to safeguard his or her integrity must always be respected. Every precaution should be taken to respect the privacy of the subject and to minimize the impact of the study on the subject's physical and mental integrity and on the personality of the subject.

7. Physicians should abstain from engaging in research projects involving human subjects unless they are satisfied that the hazards involved are believed to be predictable. Physicians

should cease any investigation if the hazards are found to outweigh the potential benefits.

8. In publication of the results of his or her research, the physician is obliged to preserve the accuracy of the results. Reports of experimentation not in accordance with the principles laid down in this Declaration should not be accepted for publication.

9. In any research on human beings, each potential subject must be adequately informed of the aims, methods, anticipated benefits and potential hazards of the study and the discomfort it may entail. He or she should be informed that he or she is at liberty to abstain from participation in the study and that he or she is free to withdraw his or her consent to participation at any time. The physician should then obtain the subject's freely-given informed consent, preferably in writing.

10. When obtaining informed consent for the research project the physician should be particularly cautious if the subject is in a dependent relationship to him or her or may consent under duress. In that case the informed consent should be obtained by a physician who is not engaged in the investigation and who is completely independent of this official relationship.

11. In case of legal incompetence, informed consent should be obtained from the legal guardian in accordance with national legislation. Where physical or mental incapacity makes it impossible to obtain informed consent, or when the subject is a minor, permission from the responsible relative replaces that of the subject in accordance with national legislation.
Whenever the minor child is in fact able to give a consent, the minor's consent must be obtained in addition to the consent of the minor's legal guardian.

12. The research protocol should always contain a statement of the ethical considerations involved and should indicate that the principles enunciated in the present Declaration are complied with.

II. MEDICAL RESEARCH COMBINED WITH PROFESSIONAL CARE
(Clinical research)

1. In the treatment of the sick person, the physician must be free to use a new diagnostic and therapeutic measure, if in his or her judgement it offers hope of saving life, reestablishing health or alleviating suffering.

2. The potential benefits, hazards and discomfort of a new method should be weighed against the advantages of the best current diagnostic and therapeutic methods.

3. In any medical study, every patient — including those of a control group, if any — should be assured of the best proven diagnostic and therapeutic method.

4. The refusal of the patient to participate in a study must never interfere with the physician-patient relationship.
5. If the physician considers it essential not to obtain informed consent, the specific reasons for this proposal should be stated in the experimental protocol for transmission to the independent committee (I, 2).
6. The physician can combine medical research with professional care, the objective being the acquisition of new medical knowledge, only to the extent that medical research is justified by its potential diagnostic or therapeutic value for the patient.

III. NON-THERAPEUTIC BIOMEDICAL RESEARCH INVOLVING HUMAN SUBJECTS
(Non-clinical biomedical research)

1. In the purely scientific application of medical research carried out on a human being, it is the duty of the physician to remain the protector of the life and health of that person on whom biomedical research is being carried out.
2. The subjects should be volunteers — either healthy persons or patients for whom the experimental design is not related to the patient's illness.
3. The investigator or the investigating team should discontinue the research if in his/her or their judgement it may, if continued, be harmful to the individual.
4. In research on man, the interest of science and society should never take precedence over considerations related to the wellbeing of the subject.

Annex 2

THE PHASES OF CLINICAL TRIALS
OF VACCINES AND DRUGS

Vaccine development

Phase I refers to the first introduction of a candidate vaccine into a human population for initial determination of its safety and biological effects, including immunogenicity. This phase may include studies of dose and route of administration, and usually involves fewer than 100 volunteers.

Phase II refers to the initial trials examining effectiveness in a limited number of volunteers (usually between 200 and 500); the focus of this phase is immunogenicity.

Phase III trials are intended for a more complete assessment of safety and effectiveness in the prevention of disease, involving a larger number of volunteers in a multicentre adequately controlled study.

Drug development

Phase I refers to the first introduction of a drug into humans. Normal volunteer subjects are usually studied to determine levels of drugs at which toxicity is observed. Such studies are followed by dose-ranging studies in patients for safety and, in some cases, early evidence of effectiveness.

Phase II investigation consists of controlled clinical trials designed to demonstrate effectiveness and relative safety. Normally, these are performed on a limited number of closely monitored patients.

Phase III trials are performed after a reasonable probability of effectiveness of a drug has been established and are intended to gather additional evidence of effectiveness for specific indications and more precise definition of drug-related adverse effects. This phase includes both controlled and uncontrolled studies.

Phase IV trials are conducted after the national drug registration authority has approved a drug for distribution or marketing. These trials may include research designed to explore a specific pharmacological effect, to establish the incidence of adverse reactions, or to determine the effects of long-term administration of a drug. Phase IV trials may also be designed to evaluate a drug in a population not studied adequately in the premarketing phases (such as children or the elderly) or to establish a new clinical indication for a drug. Such research is to be distinguished from marketing research, sales promotion studies, and routine postmarketing surveillance for adverse drug reactions in that these categories ordinarily need not be reviewed by ethical review committees (see Guideline 14).

In general, Phase I drug trials and Phase I and Phase II vaccine trials should be conducted according to the articles of the Declaration of Helsinki that refer to non-clinical research. However, some exceptions can be justified. For example, it is customary and ethically justifiable to conduct Phase I studies of highly toxic chemotherapies of cancer in patients with cancer, rather than in normal volunteers as prescribed in the Declaration of Helsinki, Article III.2. Similarly, it may be ethically justifiable to involve HIV-seropositive individuals as subjects in Phase II trials of candidate vaccines.

Phase II and Phase III drug trials should be conducted according to the articles of the Declaration of Helsinki that refer to "medical research combined with professional care (clinical research)". However, the Declaration does not provide for controlled clinical trials. Rather, it assures the freedom of the physician "to use a new diagnostic and therapeutic measure, if in his or her judgment it offers hope of saving life, reestablishing health or alleviating suffering" (Article II.1). Also in regard to Phase II and Phase III drug trials there are customary and ethically justified exceptions to the requirements of the Declaration of Helsinki. A placebo given to a control group, for example, cannot be justified by its "potential diagnostic or therapeutic value for the patient", as Article II.6 prescribes. Many other interventions and procedures characteristic of late-phase drug development have no possible diagnostic or therapeutic value for the patients and thus must be justified on other grounds; usually such justification consists of a reasonable expectation that they carry little or no risk and that they will contribute materially to the achievement of the goals of the research.

Phase III trials of vaccines do not use "a new diagnostic and therapeutic measure" that offers "hope of saving life, reestablishing health or alleviating suffering" (clinical research). Yet administration of the vaccine is intended to be a benefit to the subject rather than "the purely scientific application of medical research carried out on a human being" (non-clinical biomedical research). Thus, Phase III vaccine-trials do not conform to either of the categories defined in the Declaration of Helsinki.

APPENDIX 1

MEMBERS OF THE STEERING COMMITTEE

ABDUSSALAM, M.
Former Chairman, WHO Advisory Committee
    for Health Research for the Eastern Mediterranean
c/o Bundesgesundheitsamt
Berlin, Germany

BANKOWSKI, Z. (Secretary)
Secretary-General
Council for International Organizations of
    Medical Sciences (CIOMS)
Geneva, Switzerland

BRYANT, J.H. (Co-Chairman)
Department of Community Health Sciences
Aga Khan University
Karachi, Pakistan

CAPRON, A.M.
The Law Center
University of Southern California
Los Angeles, California, USA

COOK, R.J.
Faculty of Law
Toronto, Canada, and
Scientific and Ethical Review Group
WHO Special Programme of Research, Development and
    Research Training in Human Reproduction

DICKENS, B.M.
Faculty of Law
University of Toronto
Toronto, Canada

FLUSS, S.S.
Health Legislation
World Health Organization
Geneva, Switzerland

GALLAGHER, J.
Council for International Organizations of
    Medical Sciences (CIOMS)
Geneva, Switzerland

GILLON, R.
Imperial College of Science, Technology and Medicine
   Medical Services, and St. Mary's Hospital Medical School
University of London
London, England

GOSTIN , L.O.
WHO Collaborating Center on Health Legislation
Harvard University
Boston, Massachusetts, USA

GUTTERIDGE, F.
Council for International Organizations
   of Medical Sciences (CIOMS)
Former Director, Legal Division, World Health Organization
Geneva, Switzerland

HEYMANN, D.L.
Office of Research
Global Programme on AIDS
World Health Organization
Geneva, Switzerland

KHAN, K.S.
Department of Community Health Sciences
Aga Khan University
Karachi, Pakistan

KIMURA, R.
School of Human Sciences
Waseda University
Tokorozawa, Japan, and
Kennedy Institute of Ethics
Georgetown University
Washington, DC, USA

KOSTRZEWSKI, J.
State Institute of Hygiene
Department of Epidemiology
Warsaw, Poland

LAST, J.M.
Department of Epidemiology and Community Medicine
University of Ottawa
Ottawa, Canada

LEVINE, R.J. (Co-Chairman)
School of Medicine
Yale University
New Haven, Connecticut, USA

MARINER, W.K.
Boston University School of Public Health
Boston, Massachusetts, USA

OSUNTOKUN, B.O.
Former Chairman, WHO Global Advisory Committee
    for Health Research
Department of Medicine
University of Ibadan
Ibadan, Nigeria

QIU REN-ZONG
Institute of Philosophy
Chinese Academy of Social Sciences
Beijing, People's Republic of China

SOBERON, G.
Fundacion Mexicana para la Salud
Mexico City, Mexico

THURIAUX, M.C.
Strengthening of Epidemiological and
    Statistical Services
World Health Organization
Geneva, Switzerland

TUBIANA, M.
Former Director, Institut Gustave-Roussy
Villejuif, France

de WACHTER, M.A.M.
Institute for Bioethics
Maastricht, The Netherlands

APPENDIX 2

ADVISORS AND CONSULTANTS

BHAMARAPRAVATI, Natth
Former President
Mahidol University
Bangkok, Thailand

BYK, C.
Judge, Committee on Bioethics (Council of Europe)
Ministère de la Justice
Paris, France

CHRUSCIEL, T.
Chamber of Physicians of Poland
Warsaw, Poland

CLAYTON, A.
Fogarty International Center
National Institutes of Health
Bethesda, Maryland, USA

DUNNE, J.F.
Secretariat Committee on Research Involving Human Subjects
World Health Organization
Geneva, Switzerland

GABR, M.
Faculty of Medicine
University of Cairo
Cairo, Egypt, and
Chairman, WHO Global Adisory Committee
    for Health Research
World Health Organization
Geneva, Switzerland

GELLHORN, A.
New York State Department of Health
Albany, New York, USA

GEVERS, J.K.M.
University of Amsterdam
Amsterdam, The Netherlands

GILL, N.
Public Health Laboratory Service
Communicable Diseases Surveillance Centre
London, England

GLICK,S.
Center for Medical Education
Ben Gurion University of the Negev
Beer-Sheva, Israel

GOLDSMITH, J.
Faculty of Health Sciences
Ben Gurion University
Beer-Sheva, Israel

GUIMARAES, M.C.S.
Department of Preventive Medicine
University of Sao Paulo Medical School
Sao Paulo, Brazil

HASAN, Z.
Behavioural Science Division
Baqai Medical College
Karachi, Pakistan

JARDEL, J.-P.
Assistant Director-General
World Health Organization
Geneva, Switzerland

JEANNERET, O.
Institut de Médecine sociale et préventive
Université de Genève
Geneva, Switzerland

KANDELMAN, D.
University of Montreal
Montreal, Canada

KAPITA, B.
Hôpital Général Mama Yemo
Kinshasa, Zaïre

KELLY, R.
Stanford University
Palo Alto, California, USA

KOKKONEN, P.
Council of Europe
National Agency for Welfare and Health
Helsinki, Finland

LEGEMAATE, J.
Royal Dutch Medical Association
National Committee on AIDS Control
Maarssen, The Netherlands

LOPUKHIN, Y.
Research Institute for Physico-Chemical Medicine
Moscow, Russia

MANSOURIAN, B.G.
Office of Research and Promotion
World Health Organization
Geneva, Switzerland

MATTHEIS, R.
Senatsverwaltung für Gesundheit und Soziales
Berlin, Germany

MAURICE, N.P.
Corporate Human Research Quality Assurance Centre
Ciba-Geigy
Pharmaceutical Division
Basel, Switzerland

McCARTHY, C.R.
Former Director
Office for Protection from Research Risks
National Institutes of Health
Bethesda, Maryland, USA

MEIRIK, O.
Special Programme of Research, Development and
    Research Training in Human Reproduction
World Health Organization
Geneva, Switzerland

MILLER, J.
National Council on Bioethics in Human Research
Ottawa, Canada

NGUGI, E.
Department of Community Health and Medical
    Microbiology
University of Nairobi
Nairobi, Kenya

PORTER, J.
Department of Clinical Sciences
London School of Hygiene and Tropical Medicine
London, England

REMME, J.H.F.
Special Programme for Research and Training
    in Tropical Diseases
World Health Organization
Geneva, Switzerland

RIIS, P.
National Scientific-Ethical Committee of Denmark
Herlev, Denmark

ROSCAM-ABBING, H.
Ministry of Health
Rijswijk, The Netherlands

SARACCI, R.
International Agency for Research on Cancer
International Association of Cancer Registries
Lyon, France

SKEGG, D.C.G.
New Zealand Department of Health
Health Research Council of New Zealand
Otago, New Zealand

SOLBAKK, J.H.
The Norwegian Research Council for Science and
    the Humanities
Oslo, Norway

SUREAU, C.
Standing Committee on Ethical Aspects of Human
    Reproduction
International Federation of Gynecology
    and Obstetrics
Paris, France

de SWEEMER-BA, C.
International Development Research Centre
Dakar, Senegal

SZCZERBAN, J.
Research Promotion and Development
World Health Organization
Geneva, Switzerland

UEHARA, N.
Department of International Cooperation
    and Department of Surgery
National Medical Center
Tokyo, Japan

VILARDELL, F.
Council for International Organizations
   of Medical Sciences (CIOMS)
Escuela de Patologia Digestiva
Hospital de la Santa Cruz y San Pablo
Barcelona, Spain

WESTRIN, C.G.
Department of Social Medicine
University Hospital
Uppsala, Sweden

WIDDUS, R.
Formerly with
Global Programme on AIDS
World Health Organization
Geneva, Switzerland

WILSON, R.
Former Director
Health Sciences Division
International Development Research Centre
Ottawa, Canada

WYNEN, A.
World Medical Association
Brussels, Belgium

ZHANG JU
Department of Social Sciences
Peking Union Medical College
Beijing, People's Republic of China

ZHANG, K.-L.
Department of Epidemiology
Peking Union Medical College
Beijing, People's Republic of China

APPENDIX 3

PAPERS AND DOCUMENTS PREPARED FOR THE PROJECT

Abdussalam, M.	Ethical Review Procedures: Application of Ethical Guidelines in Non-Western Cultures[**]
Abussalam, M. and Osuntokun, B.O.	Capacity Building for Ethical Consideration of Epidemiological Studies: Perspective of Developing Countries[*]
Bhamarapravati, N.	Cultural Perspectives on Ethics and Research on Human Subjects: Vaccine Trials in Thailand[**]
Bryant, J.H.	Trends in Biomedical Ethics as Forerunners of Ethical Questions for Epidemiology[*]
Bryant, J.H.	Ethical Guidelines for Epidemiology: Precious Offering for a Troubled World[*]
Bryant, J.H. and Khan, K.S.	Epidemiology and Ethics in the Face of Scarcity[*]
Capron, A.M.	Ethical Implications of Studies in Molecular Genetics: An Emerging Issue[**]
Clayton, A.J.	Vaccine Trials: Technical Issues[*]
Dickens, B.M.	Introduction to the Draft Revised Guidelines[**]
Fluss, S.S., Simon, F. and Gutteridge, F.	Development of International Ethical Guidelines for Epidemiological Research and Practice: A Survey of Policies and Laws[*]
Gill, O. N.	Unlinked-Anonymous HIV Prevalence Monitoring[*]
Gillon, R.	Ethical Review Procedures: A Developed Countries' Perspective[**]
Gostin, L.O.	Marco-Ethical Principles for the Conduct of Research on Human Subjects: Population-Based Research and Ethics[*]
Gostin, L.O. and Jordan, L.	An Annotated Guide to Ethical Review of Research Involving Human Subjects[**]

---

* Proceedings XXVth CIOMS Conference, Geneva 1991.
** Proceedings XXVIth CIOMS Conference, Geneva 1993.

Hasan, Z.	Cultural Perspectives on Ethics and Research on Human Subjects: Eastern Mediterranean Perspective[**]
Hoffenberg, R.	Cultural Perspectives on Ethics and Research on Human Subjects: European Perspective[**]
Jardel, J.-P.	Epidemiology and Ethics: The Policymaker's Perspective[*]
Kapita, B.	Health Services for Tested Populations: Ethical Issues[*]
Kelly, R.J., Fluss, S.S. and Gutteridge, R.	The Regulation of Research on Human Subjects: A Decade of Progress[**]
Khan, K.S.	Epidemiology and Ethics: The Perspective of the Third World[*]
Khan, K.S.	Epidemiology and Ethics: The Community Perspective[*]
Kimura, R.	Cultural Perspectives on Ethics and Research on Human Subjects: Experimentation on Human Subjects in Japan[**]
Last, J.M.	Epidemiology and Ethics[*]
Levine, R.J.	Informed Consent: Some Challenges to the Universal Validity of the Western Model[*]
Levine, R.J.	Epidemiology and Ethics: The Ethicist's Perspective[*]
Levine, R.J.	Vaccine and Drug Trials — Ethical Issues[*]
Levine, R.J.	Revision of CIOMS International Ethical Guidelines for Biomedical Research Involving Human Subjects (Keynote Address of XXVIth CIOMS Conference)[**]
Mariner, W.K.	Distinguishing "Exploitable" from "Vulnerable" Populations: When Consent is not the Issue[**]
Maurice, N.P.	Obligations of Sponsors: A Sponsors' Perspective[**]
McCarthy, Ch.R.	Confidentiality: The Protection of Personal Data in Epidemiological and Clinical Research Trials[*]
McCarthy, Ch.R.	Cultural Perspectives on Ethics and Research on Human Subject: North American Perspective[**]

---

[*] Proceedings XXVth CIOMS Conference, Geneva 1991.
[**] Proceedings XXVIth CIOMS Conference, Geneva 1993.

Meirik, O. and Cook, R.	Ethical Issues in Epidemiological Research in Human Reproduction: Two Case Studies[*]
Ngugi, E.N.	Obligations of Sponsors: A Developing-Community Perspective[**]
Osuntokun, B.O.	Epidemiology and Ethics: Perspectives of Developing Countries[*]
Osuntokun, B.O.	Cultural Perspectives on Ethics and Research on Human Subjects: African Perspective[**]
Osuntokun, B.O.	Individual Informed Consent: A Perspective of Developing Countries[**]
Porter, J.D.	Ethics of Drug Trials in Developing Countries[*]
Qiu Ren-Zong	Cultural Perspectives on Ethics and Research on Human Subjects: Tension between Modern Values and Chinese Culture[**]
Soberon, G., Tarasco, M. and Kuthy, J.	Cultural Perspectives on Ethics and Research on Human Subjects: Latin American Perspective[**]
de Sweemer-Ba, C.	Individual Informed Consent: Protecting the Vulnerable[**]

---

[*] Proceedings XXVth CIOMS Conference, Geneva 1991.
[**] Proceedings XXVIth CIOMS Conference, Geneva 1993.